Diagnostic Imaging in Women's Health

OBSTETRICS AND GYNECOLOGY CLINICS OF NORTH AMERICA

www.obgyn.theclinics.com

Consulting Editor
WILLIAM F. RAYBURN, MD, MBA

March 2011 • Volume 38 • Number 1

SAUNDERS an imprint of ELSEVIER, Inc.

W.B. SAUNDERS COMPANY

A Division of Elsevier Inc.

Elsevier, Inc. • 1600 John F. Kennedy Blvd. • Suite 1800 • Philadelphia, PA 19103-2899

http://www.theclinics.com

OBSTETRICS AND GYNECOLOGY CLINICS OF NORTH AMERICA Volume 38, Number 1
March 2011 ISSN 0889-8545, ISBN-13: 978-1-4557-0887-1

Editor: Stephanie Donley
Developmental Editor: Donald Mumford

Obstetrics and Gynecology Clinics (ISSN 0889-8545) is published quarterly by Elsevier Inc., 360 Park Avenue South, New York, NY 10010-1710. Months of issue are March, June, September, and December. Periodicals postage paid at New York, NY, and additional mailing offices. Subscription price per year is $275.00 (US individuals), $474.00 (US institutions), $137.00 (US students), $331.00 (Canadian individuals), $598.00 (Canadian institutions), $201.00 (Canadian students), $402.00 (foreign individuals), $598.00 (foreign institutions), and $201.00 (foreign students). To receive student/resident rate, orders must be accompanied by name of affiliated institution, date of term, and the signature of program/residency coordinator on institution letterhead. Orders will be billed at individual rate until proof of status is received. Foreign air speed delivery is included in all *Clinics* subscription prices. All prices are subject to change without notice. POSTMASTER: Send address changes to *Obstetrics and Gynecology Clinics*, Elsevier Health Sciences Division, Subscription Customer Service, 3251 Riverport Lane, Maryland Heights, MO 63043. **Customer Service: Telephone: 1-800-654-2452 (U.S. and Canada); 314-447-8871 (outside U.S. and Canada). Fax: 314-447-8029. E-mail: journals customerservice-usa@elsevier.com (for print support); journalsonlinesupport-usa@elsevier.com (for online support).**

Reprints. For copies of 100 or more of articles in this publication, please contact the Commercial Reprints Department, Elsevier Inc., 360 Park Avenue South, New York, New York 10010-1710. Tel.: 212-633-3818; Fax: 212-462-1935; E-mail: reprints@elsevier.com.

Obstetrics and Gynecology Clinics of North America is also published in Spanish by McGraw-Hill Interamericana Editores S.A., P.O. Box 5-237, 06500, Mexico; in Portuguese by Reichmann and Affonso Editores, Rio de Janeiro, Brazil; and in Greek by Paschalidis Medical Publications, Athens, Greece.

Obstetrics and Gynecology Clinics of North America is covered in MEDLINE/PubMed (Index Medicus), Excerpta Medica, Current Concepts/Clinical Medicine, Science Citation Index, BIOSIS, CINAHL, and ISI/BIOMED.

Printed and bound by CPI Group (UK) Ltd, Croydon, CR0 4YY

Transferred to Digital Print 2011

Contributors

CONSULTING EDITOR

WILLIAM F. RAYBURN, MD, MBA
Randolph Seligman Professor and Chair, Department of Obstetrics and Gynecology;
Chief of Staff, University Hospital, University of New Mexico Health Science Center,
Albuquerque, New Mexico

AUTHORS

SUSAN J. ACKERMAN, MD
Professor, Departments of Radiology and Radiological Sciences, Medical University
of South Carolina, Charleston, South Carolina

AMNON AMIT, MD
Division of Gyneco-oncology, Rambam Health Care Campus, Faculty of Medicine,
Technion-Israel Institute of Technology, Haifa, Israel

MUNAZZA ANIS, MD
Assistant Professor, Departments of Radiology and Radiological Sciences, Medical
University of South Carolina, Charleston, South Carolina

DANIEL J. BELL, MBChB
Fellow in Body Imaging, Department of Radiology, Memorial Sloan-Kettering Cancer
Center, New York City, New York

SHWETA BHATT, MD
Department of Imaging Sciences, University of Rochester School of Medicine,
Rochester, New York

C. BOETES, MD, PhD
Professor, Department of Radiology, Maastricht University Medical Center, Maastricht,
The Netherlands

LAWRENCE A. CICCHIELLO, MD
Department of Diagnostic Radiology, Yale University School of Medicine, New Haven,
Connecticut

VIKRAM S. DOGRA, MD
Department of Imaging Sciences, University of Rochester School of Medicine,
Rochester, New York

ELIF ERGUN, MD
Instructor of Radiology, Department of Radiology, Ankara Training and Research Hospital,
Ankara, Turkey

STEPHEN FEIG, MD
Professor, Department of Radiological Sciences; Director of Breast Imaging, University
of California Irvine Medical Center, Orange, California

ULRIKE M. HAMPER, MD, MBA
Professor of Radiology and Urology Director, Division of Ultrasound, Department
of Diagnostic Radiology, The Johns Hopkins Medical Institutes, Baltimore, Maryland

ABID IRSHAD, MD
Associate Professor, Departments of Radiology and Radiological Sciences, Medical
University of South Carolina, Charleston, South Carolina

LIOR LOWENSTEIN, MD, MS
Division of Gyneco-oncology, Rambam Health Care Campus, Faculty of Medicine,
Technion-Israel Institute of Technology, Haifa, Israel

HARPREET K. PANNU, MD
Associate Attending, Department of Radiology, Memorial Sloan-Kettering Cancer Center,
New York City, New York

RAJ M. PASPULATI, MD
Assistant Professor in Radiology, Department of Radiology, University Hospitals, Case
Medical Center, Case Western Reserve University, Cleveland, Ohio

DOLORES H. PRETORIUS, MD
Professor of Radiology, Department of Radiology, University of California San Diego,
San Diego, California

ARI REISS, MD
Division of Gyneco-oncology, Rambam Health Care Campus, Faculty of Medicine,
Technion-Israel Institute of Technology, Haifa, Israel; Lady Davis Institute of Jewish
General Hospital, McGill University, Montreal, Quebec, Canada

JULIAN SCHINK, MD
Division of Gynecologic Oncology, John I. Brewer Trophoblastic Disease Center,
Northwestern University Feinberg School of Medicine, Chicago, Illinois

LESLIE M. SCOUTT, MD
Professor of Radiology and Chief, Ultrasound Service, Department of Diagnostic
Radiology, Yale University School of Medicine, New Haven, Connecticut

AHMET T. TURGUT, MD
Instructor of Radiology, Department of Radiology, Ankara Training and Research
Hospital, Ankara, Turkey

CECILE A. UNGER, MD
Resident, Department of Vincent Obstetrics and Gynecology, Massachusetts General
Hospital, Boston, Massachusetts

MILENA M. WEINSTEIN, MD
Assistant, Division of Female Pelvic Medicine and Reconstructive Surgery, Department
of Vincent Obstetrics and Gynecology, Massachusetts General Hospital, Boston,
Massachusetts

EREN D. YEH, MD
Assistant Professor of Radiology, Division of Breast Imaging, Department of Radiology,
Brigham and Women's Hospital, Dana-Farber Cancer Institute, Harvard Medical School,
Boston, Massachusetts

Contents

> This article briefly reviews the epidemiology, diagnosis, and treatment of the common gynecologic malignancies, with an emphasis on the short-comings of current clinical practice. The persistent need to achieve early diagnosis, adjust proper treatment, enhance surveillance, and improve the outcome of these patients has led to the development of new diagnostic modalities. Novel tools such as 18F-fluorodeoxyglucose PET/CT should aim at enhancing the clinician's ability to make critical decisions in treating difficult scenarios.

> Pelvic floor ultrasound is a valuable adjunct in elucidation of cause, diagnosis, and treatment of pelvic floor disorders. Three-dimensional ultrasound specifically has been shown to have many advantages over conventional imaging modalities. Proper evaluation of pelvic floor muscle function, strength, and integrity is an important component of diagnosis and treatment of pelvic floor disorders. The pelvic floor muscle training used to change the structural support and strength of muscle contraction requires clinicians to be able to conduct high-quality measurements of pelvic floor muscle function and strength. Ultrasound is a useful modality to assess the pelvic floor and its function. As practitioners become more familiar with the advantages and capabilities of ultrasound, this tool should become part of routine clinical practice in evaluation and management of pelvic floor disorders.

> Patients with gynecologic malignancies are evaluated with a combination of imaging modalities including ultrasonography (US), computed tomography (CT), and magnetic resonance (MR) imaging. US has a primary role in detecting and characterizing endometrial and adnexal pathology. CT is one of the primary modalities in staging malignancy and detecting recurrence. MR imaging is characterized by superior contrast resolution and specificity. This article reviews the role of radiologic imaging for the characterization of gynecologic masses and for staging, planning, and monitoring treatment, as well as for the assessment of tumor recurrence of the most common gynecologic malignancies.

Acute pelvic pain in women is a common presenting complaint that can result from various conditions. Because these conditions can be of gynecologic or nongynecologic origin, they may pose a challenge to the diagnostic acumen of physicians, including radiologists. A thorough workup should include clinical history, physical examination, laboratory data, and appropriate imaging studies, all of which should be available to the radiologist for evaluation. Ultrasound is the primary imaging modality in women with acute pelvic pain because of its high sensitivity, low cost, wide availability, and lack of ionizing radiation, particularly when a gynecologic disorder is suspected as the underlying cause. However, other modalities such as computed tomography (CT) and magnetic resonance imaging (MRI) may be very helpful, especially when a nongynecologic condition is suspected.

Ultrasound should be considered the first-line imaging modality of choice in women presenting with acute or chronic pelvic pain of suspected gynecologic or obstetric origin because many, if not most, gynecologic/obstetric causes of pelvic pain are easily diagnosed on ultrasound examination. Since the clinical presentation of gynecologic causes of pelvic pain overlaps with gastrointestinal and genitourinary pathology, referral to CT or MRI, especially in pregnant patients, should be considered if the US examination is nondiagnostic.

Vaginal bleeding is the most common cause of emergency care in the first trimester of pregnancy and accounts for the majority of premenopausal bleeding cases. Ultrasound evaluation combined with a quantitative beta human chorionic gonadotropin test is an established diagnostic tool to assess these patients. Spontaneous abortion because of genetic abnormalities is the most common cause of vaginal bleeding; ectopic pregnancy and gestational trophoblastic disease are other important causes and in all patients presenting with first trimester bleeding, ectopic pregnancy should be suspected and excluded, as it is associated with significant maternal morbidity and mortality. A thorough knowledge of the normal sonographic appearance of intrauterine gestation is essential to understand the manifestations of an abnormal gestation. Arteriovenous malformation of the uterus is a rare but important cause of vaginal bleeding in the first trimester, as it has to be differentiated from the more common retained products of conception, with which it is often mistaken.

Breast cancer is the most common cancer in women. One in 8 women develops breast cancer and approximately 30% of all affected women die of the disease. By performing a nationwide screening program in the Netherlands, a mortality reduction of 1.2% annually was achieved. The screening program is for women between the ages of 50 and 75 years; however, women with an increased risk for developing breast cancer are mostly younger. The role of MRI in this particular group of women has been described in different studies. MRI of the breast in this group of women has a higher sensitivity than mammography, but the highest sensitivity is reached by the combination of these two imaging modalities.

Eren D. Yeh

Breast magnetic resonance (MR) is highly sensitive in the detection of invasive breast malignancies. As technology improves, as interpretations and reporting by radiologists become standardized through the development of guidelines by expert consortiums, and as scientific investigation continues, the indications and uses of breast MR as an adjunct to mammography continue to evolve. This article discusses the current clinical indications for breast MR including screening for breast cancer, diagnostic indications for breast MR, and MR guidance for interventional procedures.

Stephen Feig

Screening mammography performed annually on all women beginning at age 40 years has reduced breast cancer deaths by 30% to 50%. The cost per year of life saved is well within the range for other commonly accepted medical interventions. Various studies have estimated that reduction in treatment costs through early screening detection may be 30% to 100% or more of the cost of screening. Magnetic resonance imaging (MRI) screening is also cost-effective for very high-risk women, such as BRCA carriers, and others at 20% or greater lifetime risk. Further studies are needed to determine whether MRI is cost-effective for those at moderately high (15%–20%) lifetime risk. Future technical advances could make MRI more cost-effective than it is today. Automated whole-breast ultrasonography will probably prove cost-effective as a supplement to mammography for women with dense breasts.

THE CLINICS ARE NOW AVAILABLE ONLINE!

Access your subscription at:
www.theclinics.com

Foreword

Diagnostic Imaging in Women's Health

This unique issue of the *Obstetrics and Gynecology Clinics of North America* deals with updates on diagnostic imaging techniques that apply to women's health. Such techniques can be integral cornerstones of gynecology since most patients, at one time or another, undergo some form of imaging to enhance clinical diagnosis in directing their care. As the availability of diagnostic imaging tools has increased and become more diverse and sophisticated, information obtained from these techniques for the obstetrician-gynecologist has added not only more detailed morphologic, but also functional diagnostic information.

The obstetrician-gynecologist's use and understanding of diagnostic ultrasound varies, yet CT, MRI, and now the newer PET studies may seem mysterious and completely beyond their realm. Common questions are "what type of study should be ordered for this clinical condition," and "how should the findings be used in clinical management decisions?" Additionally, cost-benefit issues being faced by accountable care organizations are continually on the minds of providers and patients alike.

Given the quality of recent past articles in radiology-related *Clinics* publications and their relevance to women's health, the publishers of this series and I selected articles from recent issues of those *Clinics* to be presented here for the benefit of our readership. In this issue, the authors provide diagnostic imaging topics pertinent to the obstetrician-gynecologist that the reader may not have the inclination to read because of the nature of publication specialization. When the clinician adds other medical information to the thoughtfulness behind diagnostic reporting, their perspective may be enhanced by the differential diagnosis that the imaging specialist may face.

Examples of gynecologic conditions for which an ultrasound, MRI, CT, or PET study may be relevant would include perimenopausal bleeding, pelvic pain, pelvic floor disorders, assessment of gynecologic malignancies, and breast cancer evaluation. Dr Paspulati and colleagues demonstrate a wonderful visual review of the most common classic sonographic findings for the patient with perimenopausal bleeding. Since pelvic pain affects 20–50% of all females, it is likely that they will have some type of initial ultrasound examination. Dr Ackerman, Dr Cicchiello, and their respective coauthors present findings in patients with pelvic pain due to nongynecologic and gynecologic etiologies. As the subspecialty of urogynecology has added an entirely new area of pelvic floor imaging, the patient with incontinence symptoms has increasingly become able to receive treatment-altering imaging, as reported here by Dr Unger and colleagues.

Radiologic assessment for gynecologic malignancies is nicely reviewed by Dr Bell and Dr Pannu. Dr Amit and colleagues discuss the remarkable increase in the number of articles in F-fluorodeoxyglucose (FDG)-PET and why use of this modality in gynecologic cancer assessment has piqued the interest of clinicians. Our patients who anxiously return from their various breast imaging studies are better served with an improved understanding of what each type of study distinctly offers. Dr Yeh and Dr Boetes provide

Obstet Gynecol Clin N Am 38 (2011) xi–xii
doi:10.1016/j.ogc.2011.02.010
0889-8545/11/$ – see front matter © 2011 Elsevier Inc. All rights reserved.

detailed indications and standards of breast MRI, especially among high-risk patients. Finally, Dr Feig addresses a very important cost analysis of all the above imaging modalities for breast cancer screening.

It is rewarding for me to interact with repeat contributors and to again call upon their expertise and knowledge. I am grateful to the dedicated individuals for their willingness, even eagerness, to update their contributions for this special issue dedicated to obstetrician-gynecologists. Special thanks go to Stephanie Donley, our editor, for her continued help and support and to Rebecca Hall, PhD, at the Women's Imaging Center, Department of Obstetrics and Gynecology at the University of New Mexico for her assistance in helping me select these articles that would have the most appeal to our readership.

William F. Rayburn, MD, MBA
Department of Obstetrics and Gynecology
University of New Mexico School of Medicine
MSC 10 5580; 1 University of New Mexico
Albuquerque, NM 87131-0001, USA

E-mail address:
wrayburn@salud.unm.edu

PET/CT in Gynecologic Cancer: Present Applications and Future Prospects—A Clinician's Perspective

Amnon Amit, MD[a],*, Julian Schink, MD[b], Ari Reiss, MD[a,c],
Lior Lowenstein, MD, MS[a]

KEYWORDS

- ^{18}F-Fluorodeoxyglucose PET • Gynecologic cancer
- Cross-sectional imaging • Best practice

Providing the proper care for patients with gynecologic malignancies has always been a challenge for clinicians. The persistent need to achieve early diagnosis, adjust proper treatment, enhance surveillance, and improve the outcome of these patients has led to the development of new diagnostic modalities. The last decade witnessed great progress in the use of cross-sectional imaging techniques, such as ultrasonography (US), computed tomography (CT), and magnetic resonance (MR) imaging. These imaging modalities are able to demonstrate anatomic details and morphologic changes, but often fail to discriminate between benign and malignant lesions. The functional information obtained from ^{18}F-fluorodeoxyglucose (FDG) PET exhibits the high uptake of glucose by malignant cells, but lacks anatomic landmarks. The fusion of PET with CT combines the advantages of these 2 modalities, allowing the anatomic localization of metabolic abnormalities in the female genital tract and beyond in patients with disseminated disease.

The literature on FDG-PET in gynecologic malignancies between the years 2000 and 2009 reveals a significant increase in the number of articles that have been published. Whereas in 2003 only one article was published, more than 70 articles were listed in

A version of this article was previously published in *PET Clinics* 5:4.
[a] Division of Gyneco-oncology, Rambam Health Care Campus, Faculty of Medicine, Technion-Israel Institute of Technology, Haifa 9602, Israel
[b] Division of Gynecologic Oncology, John I. Brewer Trophoblastic Disease Center, Northwestern University Feinberg School of Medicine, 250 East Superior Street, Suite 5-2168, Chicago, IL, USA
[c] Lady Davis Institute of Jewish General Hospital, McGill University, Montreal, Quebec, Canada
* Corresponding author. Department of Obstetrics and Gynecology, Rambam Medical Center, 9 Ha'Aliya Street, Haifa 31096, Israel.
E-mail address: a_amit@rambam.health.gov.il

Obstet Gynecol Clin N Am 38 (2011) 1–21
doi:10.1016/j.ogc.2011.02.001
0889-8545/11/$ – see front matter © 2011 Elsevier Inc. All rights reserved.

2009, the vast majority reporting on the use of PET/CT. An attempt to obtain similar information concerning CT and MR imaging divulges a constant average number of 90 articles each year. This increase reflects the clinicians' growing interest in this promising modality, which attempts and is often successful in overcoming some limitations of former conventional diagnostic approach.

This article briefly reviews the epidemiology, diagnosis, and treatment of the common gynecologic malignancies, with an emphasis on the shortcomings of current clinical practice.

CERVICAL CANCER
Epidemiology

Cervical cancer is one of the leading causes of death among women with gynecologic malignancies[1] and the median age of diagnosis is approximately 48 years in the United States. Recent studies indicate that human papilloma virus (HPV) infection is the main cause of this disease.[2] High-risk viral subtypes (mainly types 16 and 18) increase the risk of developing high-grade cervical dysplasia and cancer. Important risk factors include increased number of sexual partners, early age at first coitus, low socioeconomic status, compromised immune system, smoking, and diethylstilbestrol exposure. Most cervical cancers are squamous in histology, with adenocarcinoma being the second most common histologic type.

Prevention and Screening

Two HPV vaccines have recently been approved by the United States Food and Drug Administration. These vaccines were developed against the viral subtypes 16 and 18, which are responsible for 75% of cervical cancers. Recent studies have demonstrated that these vaccines are highly immunogenic and reduce rates of cervical intraepithelial neoplasia significantly, with an efficacy near 100% in women previously not exposed to these viral subtypes. The recommendations from the United States Centers for Disease Control and Prevention and from other medical authorities are to begin vaccination at the age of 11 or even as early as 9 years.[3]

Because invasive cervical cancer has a preinvasive phase (cervical intraepithelial neoplasia), screening is an effective tool in risk reduction. Regular Pap smear screening, as done in the United States, has dramatically reduced the incidence and mortality of this disease. Although sensitivity for a single examination is relatively low (50%–70%), repeat examinations (every 2–3 years) may at least partly overcome this limitation. It has also been suggested that the identification of high-risk types of HPV has improved the sensitivity and specificity of the Pap smear test in certain circumstances, such as when having atypical cells or atypical glandular cells of undetermined significance (ASCUS/AGUS). However, HPV typing as a screening modality has yet to be evaluated, mainly for its cost effectiveness.

Natural Course of the Disease

Following a preinvasive stage, located mainly in the squamo-columnar junction, the cancer invades the cervical stroma and then spreads by direct invasion into the parametrium, uterus, and vagina. As the disease advances, the tumor spreads through lymphatic channels toward the pelvic, para-aortic, and supraclavicular lymph nodes. Hematogenic spread to the lungs, liver, or any other distant organ may be observed at any stage, although it is unlikely to occur in the early stages of the disease.

Diagnosis

Following an abnormal Pap test, women are evaluated with colposcopy and directed biopsies. In the case of high-grade intraepithelial lesions (HGSIL) or in cases of suspected pathologic Pap smear along with suboptimal colposcopy, conization of the cervix is recommended.

Staging

In contrast to endometrial and ovarian cancer, cervical cancer is staged clinically, because of the prevalence of the disease in underserved countries where technology is not available. **Table 1** summarizes the International Federation for Gynecology and Obstetrics (FIGO) clinical staging, treatment options, and 5-year survival rates for every stage. Staging procedures include physical examination, chest radiograph, intravenous pyelogram (IVP), cystoscopy, and rectoscopy. However, most medical centers employ cross-sectional imaging techniques such as US, CT, MR imaging, and FDG-PET/CT to overcome the limitations of traditional diagnostic methods. Surgical staging with lymphadenectomy is more accurate than clinical staging, but is controversial among gynecologic oncologists, as there is no proof of any survival benefits of the procedure, especially with microscopic nodal disease.[4] Using new diagnostic modalities or any information obtained from surgical procedures will not change staging, but may lead to treatment adjustment.

Treatment

Treatment in the early stages of the disease includes surgery or radiotherapy. In locally advanced disease, radiotherapy is combined with chemotherapy, and in metastatic disease the treatment is chemotherapy.[5–7] Patients with early (Stage IA) squamous cell cancer (microinvasive) and no lymph-vascular space invasion (LVSI) can be treated with simple, extrafascial hysterectomy. Stage IB to IIA disease is usually treated with radical hysterectomy and pelvic lymphadenectomy, but can be treated with primary radiation therapy with similar outcomes.[8] However, clinicians and patients alike tend to opt for surgery because of the possible complications of radiation, including loss of ovarian function, bowel stricture, and fistula formation.

Young females with early disease desiring future fertility can be treated with conization of the cervix alone or with radical trachalectomy, which removes the cervix,

Table 1
FIGO clinical staging, treatment, and 5-year survival for cervical cancer

FIGO Stage Criteria	Treatment Options	5-Year Survival
O. Carcinoma in situ	Conization, TAH	96%–100%
IA. Microscopic lesions	Conization, modified hysterectomy[a]	92%–94%
IB1. Macroscopic lesion ≤4 cm	RH, RTL, XRT/Chemo	80.7%
IB2. Macroscopic lesion ≥4 cm	RH, XRT/Chemo	79%
IIA. Vaginal involvement	RH, XRT/Chemo	76%
IIB. Parametrial involvement	XRT/Chemo	73.3%
IIIA. Lower one-third of vagina	XRT/Chemo	50.5%
IIIB. Side wall extension and/or hydronephrosis	XRT/Chemo	46%
IVA. Adjacent organ involvement	XRT/Chemo	29%
IVB. Distant metastasis	Chemo, palliative XRT	22%

Abbreviations: Chemo, chemotherapy; RH, radical hysterectomy; RTL, radical trachelectomy; TAH, total abdominal hysterectomy; XRT, radiotherapy.
[a] Individualization by patient's age and fertility desire.

parametrial tissue, and upper vagina while preserving the uterus for future child-bearing. A permanent cervical cerclage and assisted reproductive technologies are required in this setting. Prognosis appears to be acceptable in this group regarding survival, recurrence, and pregnancy outcomes. However, these patients need close follow-up so as to exclude recurrence.[4,9]

When the cancer has progressed beyond the cervix, but is still limited to the pelvis (Stages IIB through IVA), primary chemo-radiotherapy is used. Radiation therapy is delivered by a combination of tele- and brachytherapy to deliver an adequate dose to the cervix, parametrium, and pelvic lymph nodes. Hysterectomy may be performed after radiation therapy in patients with residual disease. However, the morbidity caused by combining surgery and chemo-radiotherapy must be taken into consideration in such cases. Postoperative chemo-radiotherapy is recommended for patients who have had a radical hysterectomy with the following risk factors for final pathology: parametrial involvement, close or positive vaginal margins, positive lymph nodes, and certain tumor characteristics such as LVSI, tumor size, and deep stromal invasion.[7] Distant metastatic cervical cancer (Stage IVB) has a poor prognosis and is palliated with chemotherapy, which provides a limited survival benefit. The combination of cisplatin and topotecan is currently the treatment of choice.[10]

Recurrence

Recurrent cervical cancer has a dismal prognosis if not limited to the pelvis. If the recurrent disease is limited to the central pelvis without other metastases, and if no pelvic side-wall involvement is identified, long-term survival may be achieved. Radiation therapy is recommended for locally confined recurrent disease in patients who have not already undergone this treatment. In previously radiated patients, pelvic exenteration (anterior, posterior, or total) offers survival rates of 20% to 60%.[11] With nonresectable disease, overall survival is less than 1 year.

Special Considerations and Unmet Clinical Needs in the Evaluation and Treatment of Patients with Cervical Cancer

This section updates and summarizes the clinician's needs in specific areas.

Staging and evaluation of newly diagnosed patients with cervical cancer

The main challenge in this group of patients is to choose the best treatment in terms of survival benefits with the lowest toxicity. Following initial diagnosis, this group is usually divided into 3 subgroups.

Patients with early disease: Stages I to IIA These patients may be treated by either radical hysterectomy or pelvic radiotherapy, with a similar overall survival. However, many patients who undergo radical hysterectomy are subsequently referred to radiotherapy secondary to failure of clinical and imaging modalities, despite the fact it can result in long-term toxicity with no survival benefits.

All current modalities that are expected to guide surgeons in assessing invasion into the cervical stroma and early parametrial involvement are characterized by a relatively low sensitivity in the early stages of the disease.[12] Clinicians are therefore unable to avoid bimodality treatment. Thus, even though the disease is confined to the cervix, these patients will be referred to radiotherapy to reduce the chances of recurrence.

Another main concern is pelvic and para-aortic lymph node (PALN) status. Positive pelvic lymph nodes are the most important prognostic factor, and radical hysterectomy may be abandoned if suspected positive lymph nodes are detected in frozen-section pathology. FDG-PET/CT, with its high specificity, may allow clinicians to avoid unnecessary surgery and to refer patients to chemo-radiotherapy, making it the imaging procedure of choice in evaluating this group of patients. These patients will be closely followed secondary to a high probability of recurrence.

Semiquantitative measurements of the degree of FDG uptake using maximum standardized uptake value (SUV$_{max}$) was recently studied in several aspects of cervical cancer. Further experience is needed to estimate the use of this modality in characterizing the aggressiveness of a tumor and in predicting stromal invasion and pelvic lymph node metastasis.[13]

Patients with locally advanced disease These patients represent, according to clinical staging, 15% to 30% of patients with pelvic disease who will eventually have lymph node metastases.[4] Patients with locally advanced disease are usually treated with chemo-radiotherapy. The goal in treating these patients is to exclude extrapelvic disease and to achieve the best definition for a radiation field. Positive PALN may alter the radiation field and lead to a different chemotherapy regimen. Disseminated disease may change the approach of treatment in the direction of palliative care and obviate the need for radiation in end-stage patients.

Several studies have demonstrated the superiority of FDG imaging over CT and MR imaging in detecting metastatic lesions in patients with advanced disease.[14–17] PET/CT provides better localization and definition of metastatic sites.[18] The sensitivity of FDG-PET is in direct correlation with the stage of disease and probably relates to the volume of the tumor present in affected nodes.[19] For patients with advanced disease, the sensitivity of FDG-PET/CT in detecting PALN metastases is 95%.[17,20,21] A limitation of some these studies is that they did not use histopathology as a gold standard, because most patients did not undergo a surgical procedure. Other drawbacks are related to the fact that PET/CT results were not always translated into survival benefits, and also that most studies include a relatively small number of patients. However, the superiority of PET/CT over CT and MR imaging has emerged from many studies in different medical centers. Assuming that patients with advanced disease will have a worse prognosis, the accuracy of these results is often dependent on a relatively long-term follow-up, which may partially overcome the lack of pathology results. Up-to-date PET/CT results are an indicator of its importance as a tool to be used in evaluating patients with locally advanced disease. Future efforts should focus on improving the accuracy of disease detection through the fusion of PET with another modality, such as MR imaging, or through the use of other metabolic agents.

Patients with metastatic cervical cancer When newly diagnosed, these patients have a poor prognosis (see **Table 1**). Treatment is primarily palliative, with the goal being control of symptoms. Some studies have demonstrated the ability to detect, characterize, and locate lesions in supraclavicular and mediastinal lymph nodes, lungs, bones, peritoneum, omentum, and liver.[22–24] Because metastatic disease in newly diagnosed patients is uncommon, comparative studies demonstrating the additional value of PET/CT are scarce. Clinicians may gain some experience from recurrent studies that enable one to demonstrate the value of PET/CT in restaging these patients and specifically assessing distant lesions.

Radiotherapy planning

Radiotherapy in patients with cervical cancer aims at destroying malignant lesions by delivering maximal doses to a specific location while attempting to avoid the radiation of healthy tissues. Because radiotherapy can cause severe toxicity, there is a true clinical need to define the borders between healthy and malignant tissue in the primary tumor. Having a diagnostic modality that can provide this information can be very helpful for clinicians in their efforts to improve radiotherapy planning and outcome.

As previously noted, PET/CT has been shown to have the best accuracy in detecting disease in lymph nodes and distant lesions, and therefore is the most useful tool for directing radiotherapists to the affected sites. Many recent studies have been conducted using FDG-PET/CT to demonstrate the actively metabolic borders of the primary cervical tumor and distant active lesions. According to these studies, PET/CT images should be transferred to the radiotherapy treatment planning system so that the contour of normal organs can be delivered from the CT portion and metastatic active sites can be contoured from the PET component. Subsequent radiation doses at the prescribed volume can be planned using the radiotherapy treatment planning software.[19] Additional studies need to be conducted in the future to establish the role and integration of PET/CT in radiotherapy treatment planning systems.

Determination of prognostic pretreatment parameters and response to therapy

Assessing a patient's prognosis is of great importance, as it may change treatment planning to improve outcome. Prognosis can be determined by pretreatment parameters and by response to treatment, which may dictate additional therapy and/or a different follow-up policy (see **Table 1**). Before the introduction of PET/CT, prognosis was estimated by the patient's age, stage, grade, presence of positive pelvic and PALN, and by other tumor indices, such as tumor volume and lymph and vascular space involvement.[18]

In many medical centers, PET/CT is now routinely performed for pretreatment evaluation and prognosis determination. Experience gained over the last few years indicates that PET/CT is of additional value in determining the patient's prognosis and treatment response, mainly due to its high accuracy in detecting affected lymph nodes. Moreover, studies have shown that evaluating a patient's prognosis using SUV_{max} values in primary tumors and assessing the metabolic activity 3 months after completion of radiotherapy may provide important information for significantly improving the outcome.[13,25–28] Brooks and colleagues[26] evaluated the role of PET/CT in detecting symptomatic versus asymptomatic recurrent cervical cancer. Their findings demonstrated a significant survival benefit in asymptomatic patients with recurrent disease detected by PET/CT as compared with symptomatic patients.[26] This study and others have led some medical centers to implement PET/CT as a routine diagnostic imaging modality for patients with cervical cancer.

Patient follow-up and early detection of recurrent disease

Surveillance protocols of patients with cervical cancer usually consist of a physical examination, Pap smear, and a chest radiograph performed at different intervals according to risk factors. However, it is uncommon to detect a symptomatic patient using this surveillance policy. Pelvic examination and vaginal or cervical cytology are of limited use because of radiation-associated changes. Obliteration of the vaginal vault is common, and parametrial fibrosis increases the difficulties of assessing the normal anatomy.[29–31] Evaluation of lymph node status using a pelvic examination is impossible, making it highly unlikely that recurrence of the disease will be detected in asymptomatic patients.

As already noted, the implementation of routine CT scans has not been shown to contribute significantly to outcome. MR imaging shows better results than CT, but is not good enough to be used as a routine imaging modality.[32] Morice and colleagues[33] showed that using CT and MR imaging during routine follow-up did not change the survival rates of patients with cervical cancer. These limitations increase the clinician's need for a better diagnostic modality that allows detection of asymptomatic recurrence. Early detection of central pelvic recurrence may result in salvage surgery (ie, pelvic exenteration) with curative intent and survival benefits.

In summary, FDG-PET/CT meets the clinical need for an effective imaging modality in the early detection of recurrent disease, and provides better localization and definition of metastatic sites in patients with advanced disease. The evidence supports that PET/CT be used for routine follow-up purposes and can provide a better outcome. However, surveillance intervals should be further investigated to define the survival benefits and cost effectiveness.

OVARIAN CANCER
Epidemiology

Ovarian cancer is the sixth most common malignancy in women worldwide and the second most common gynecologic malignancy, accounting for about 21,500 new cases and 15,000 deaths a year in the United States. The lifetime risk of developing ovarian cancer is about 1.6%.[34] Despite strenuous research and screening efforts, this malignancy still constitutes a major diagnostic and therapeutic problem.

Epithelial tumors account for about 90% of malignant ovarian tumors.[35] Less common types are germ cell or stromal tumors. Commonly known risk factors are age, family history, genetics, nulliparity, early menarche, and late menopause.[36] More than two-thirds of ovarian cancers present during the postmenopausal period, at a median age of 63 years.[37] Family history is recognized as a significant risk factor, with women whose mothers had ovarian cancer carrying a 7% risk of developing the disease themselves.[38]

The most common genetic mutations associated with ovarian cancer are BRCA-1 and BRCA-2, commonly found among Ashkenazi Jews. The average cumulative risk for ovarian cancer by age 70 years is 39% (18%–54%) in BRCA-1 mutation carriers and 11% (2.4%–19%) in BRCA-2 mutation carriers. Lynch syndrome (hereditary nonpolyposis colon cancer syndrome) is another genetic entity associated with an increase in the lifetime risk for ovarian cancer of up to 10% to 15%.[39] The use of oral contraceptives,[40] parity, and bilateral oopherectomy are known to be protective factors against the development of ovarian cancer.

Diagnosis

The main challenges of the primary practitioner in the early diagnosis of ovarian cancer are the lack of specific early signs and symptoms and the absence of effective screening programs. About 75% of cases are diagnosed at an advanced stage, leading to high morbidity and poor survival rates.[41,42] Most commonly, the tumor spreads into the peritoneal cavity. Lymphatic and hematogenic spread are less common routes of dissemination for this type of tumor.[43,44]

The majority of patients present with vague and nonspecific symptoms, such as abdominal discomfort and distention. In a more advanced stage patients may present with gastrointestinal symptoms secondary to bowel obstruction. Tumor metastases to liver parenchyma and extra-abdominal organs, as well as pleural effusion, are relatively uncommon and are more characteristic of late stages of the disease.

Diagnosis relies on the detection of pelvic and abdominal masses, and ascites.[45,46] Patients with suspected ovarian cancer undergo a thorough physical examination, including abdominal palpation and bimanual vaginal examination. In most cases, an adnexal mass is palpated. Other abdominal masses may be recognized in advanced cases. Serum levels of CA125 (a glycoprotein tumor marker) can be useful in distinguishing malignant from benign pelvic masses, especially in postmenopausal patients. The combination of an adnexal mass with an elevated serum level of CA125 >200 IU/mL in a postmenopausal woman was found to have a positive predictive value of 97% for ovarian cancer diagnosis.[47–49]

Imaging modalities are commonly used for diagnosing abdominal masses and differentiating them from ovarian cancer. Common sonographic signs related to ovarian cancer are complex ovarian masses, irregular cysts with papillae, low-resistance flow in ovarian blood vessels as measured by Doppler, and ascites.[50] CT is commonly used for the evaluation of disease spread and for the differentiation of ovarian cancer from other malignancies.[51]

Treatment

The standard treatment of ovarian cancer includes cytoreductive surgery and chemotherapy drugs. The goal of surgery is to remove all tumor load, so-called optimal debulking.[52–56] During surgery, a total hysterectomy, bilateral salpingo-oophorectomy, and infracolic omentectomy are performed. Peritoneal biopsies and retroperitoneal lymph node sampling are also performed as part of the staging process.

To obtain optimal debulking, any macroscopically visible tumor needs to be surgically removed.[57,58] The significance of optimal debulking is its association with prognosis of ovarian cancer.[59,60] Patients whose tumor has been completely resected to a state of no macroscopic residual disease are found to have significantly better survival rates than patients who still have remaining macroscopic tumor.[60] In some cases, surgical removal of the entire tumor may not be feasible due to poor patient condition, stage IV disease, or high metastatic tumor load.[61,62]

Neoadjuvant chemotherapy, consisting of 3 to 4 courses of intravenous chemotherapy administered before the surgical procedure, is commonly used to reduce the tumor burden and allow optimal debulking. A recent large prospective, randomized, controlled multicenter study conducted by the gynecologic cancer group (EORTC-GCG) demonstrated that in cases of advanced ovarian tumors, neoadjuvant chemotherapy followed by interval debulking surgery may result in similar survival rates as those for standard primary debulking surgery followed by adjuvant chemotherapy.[63–65] Adjuvant chemotherapy is needed in cases of tumor capsule penetration and beyond. Nowadays, different chemotherapy drugs are used for treating ovarian cancer. Current first-line chemotherapy for epithelial tumors is the combination of paclitexal plus a platinum analogue for 6 to 8 cycles.[66–68] Ongoing research in chemotherapy for ovarian cancer is driven by both drug companies and gyneco-oncologist research groups, such as the gynecologic oncology group (GOG).

Prognosis

Prognosis of ovarian cancer is highly dependent on tumor stage, histologic type and differentiation, surgical outcome (optimal debulking vs nonoptimal debulking), and other comorbidity factors. A study by Heintz and colleagues[69] demonstrated that survival rates are highly associated with the surgical stage of the disease at diagnosis. The approximate 5-year survival rate of patients is: Stage I disease, 90%; Stage II, 65%; Stage III, 40%; and Stage IV, 18%.[69] Although the overall response rate with primary therapy is about 80%, the majority of patients will ultimately relapse and die of the disease within 5 years of diagnosis.[70,71] If the disease recurs within 6 months following treatment, it is considered to be platinum-resistant. Chemotherapy for platinum-resistant patients includes pegylated and liposomal drugs, doxorubicin, Hycamtin (topotecan hydrochloride), and gemcitabine. A second-look operation is performed for the evaluation of treatment response. Its current use is mainly for research purposes.

Staging

In recent years, FDG-PET/CT has been recognized as a new modality that can potentially assist in the diagnosis of tumor spread and in the detection of early recurrence of the disease.[72–74] Current screening algorithms, using the measurement of CA125 serum levels and ultrasound imaging of the ovaries, have yielded low positive predictive values, and their ability to lower the stage of disease at the time of diagnosis remains questionable.[75] PET/CT might have a potential role in improving the screening algorithms. There are sporadic case reports describing the detection of early-stage ovarian cancer using PET/CT.[76,77] Risum and colleagues[73] suggested the use of PET/CT in cases who present with elevated CA125 serum levels, combined with a suspected ovarian mass seen on US. The sensitivity and specificity of PET/CT in such cases was 100% and 92%, respectively.

Prevention and Screening

Early diagnosis is probably the key point in reducing the mortality and morbidity associated with ovarian cancer. Patients diagnosed at an early stage (Stage I) have a significantly better diagnosis than patients diagnosed at a late stage (Stages III and IV), with 5-year survival rates estimated at 90% and 25%, respectively.[78] Intensive research is currently ongoing to identify additional markers and a cost-effective screening strategy. Several screening programs using ultrasound and CA125 serum levels demonstrated relatively earlier stage detection, but failed to show survival benefits.

Evidence suggests that screening programs are appropriate for women with a family history of ovarian cancer or familial ovarian cancer syndromes. Previous research has evaluated the role of screening programs in the early detection of ovarian cancer in high-risk populations.[79,80] In one study, 4 years of screening with CA125 serum levels and transvaginal ultrasound revealed a sensitivity of 40% and a specificity of 99% in a series of 312 women 35 years or older, and carriers for BRCA-1 or BRCA-2 mutations.[81]

Screening recommendations for higher-risk women depend on whether there is a known or suspected hereditary cancer syndrome. Diagnostic modalities such as CT and MR imaging have been tested and have not demonstrated any advantage in this regard. Many other tumor markers are under investigation, but as yet lack clinical application. The role of PET/CT has not been thoroughly explored, but possible limitations for the use of this modality for screening are its high cost and lack of specificity.

Once the disease has been diagnosed, there is a question regarding the additive role of additional imaging modalities in treatment planning.[74,82] The utility of CT in determining complete resection of the tumor in advanced cases is of limited value.[83] Several studies have investigated the incremental value of preoperative PET/CT to estimate the feasibility of achieving optimal debulking in an advanced disease stage.[74] Previous studies have also demonstrated stage migration when comparing PET/CT with CT.[73] However, PET/CT is still not being routinely used preoperatively for such purposes.

Following the diagnosis of ovarian tumor, preoperative evaluation should be aimed to achieve several objectives:

1. Rule out other primary tumors with metastases to the ovaries (mainly of breast or gastrointestinal origin).

2. Estimate the feasibility of achieving optimal debulking. Once it is determined that complete resection of the tumor is not possible, neoadjuvant treatment may be administered. Although the neoadjuvant approach has not been proven to increase survival rates, it may have a positive impact on quality of life.
3. Gain better knowledge concerning the location of any metastasis to assign the ideal team for surgery (urologist, general surgeon, and so forth).

Recurrence

Patient follow-up and evaluation for recurrence of the disease is done mainly by periodic physical examination, repeated testing of CA125 serum levels, and CT if needed.[84] The add-on value of early detection of disease recurrence is controversial, with recent studies demonstrating that apart from the increase in the number of chemotherapy courses administered, there was no added benefit in terms of survival time and quality of life in cases where early recurrence was detected. Based on these data, it is not clear whether tests with higher sensitivity are clinically effective in the earlier detection of disease recurrence.

When disease recurs, the clinician needs to know whether it is a localized recurrence or disseminated disease. This information is crucial in making the decision to attempt a second debulking. If the disease is disseminated, the clinician needs a reliable method for monitoring treatment results in order to avoid unnecessary chemotherapy if it fails to achieve a response. PET/CT appears to play a potentially important role in early detection of recurrent ovarian cancer and, if detected, in determining whether it is localized or disseminated.

The differentiation between a borderline and a full-blown tumor is also highly significant. A borderline tumor can usually be treated by unilateral oopherectomy. Clinical evaluation and presurgical assessment can assist in better planning of surgery. Neither CT nor US are good tools for differentiating between borderline and malignant tumors. Risum and colleagues[73] have reported normal metabolic results in all their 7 cases diagnosed with borderline tumors.

Other than early primary diagnosis of the disease, early detection of tumor recurrence and the differentiation between borderline and full-blown tumors are among the most common challenging issues in the management of ovarian cancer today. Cumulative research in gynecology is required to determine the role of PET/CT in helping to resolve them.

ENDOMETRIAL CANCER
Epidemiology

Endometrial cancer, a tumor of the endometrial lining of the uterine corpus, is the most common genital tract cancer, and the fourth most common malignancy occurring in women living in developed countries worldwide.[85] This disease trails only breast, colon, and lung cancer, with an estimated 136,000 cases per year. Endometrial cancer is associated with excess estrogen levels, either from endogenous or exogenous sources. Obesity and diabetes are linked to increased levels of circulating unbound endogenous estrogen, and with the epidemic of obesity, the incidence of this cancer is expected to increase.

Background and Natural Course of the Disease

The overall prognosis for endometrial cancer is 75%, with greater than 90% disease-free survival for women with Stage I disease. The good outcome seen in this malignancy reflects that early diagnosis usually occurs when women report abnormal vaginal bleeding, either postmenopausal or heavy intermenstrual bleeding. The tumor is generally confined to the uterus at the time of diagnosis, with only 10% to 20% of surgically staged patients having lymph node metastases at the time of surgery.[85] The staging system for endometrial cancer is defined by FIGO. The recent revision of this staging system in 2009 (**Box 1**), is based on surgical staging that ideally includes total hysterectomy, bilateral salpingo-oophorectomy, pelvic and PALN dissection, and assessment of peritoneal cytology. Lymph node metastases and survival are predicted by depth of myometrial invasion, tumor grade, histology, and tumor size.[86]

Diagnosis and Pretreatment Assessment

The diagnosis of endometrial cancer is usually the result of an office endometrial biopsy or uterine dilatation and curettage (D&C), with or without hysteroscopy, performed under sedation in a surgical suite. These procedures are indicated if a woman complains of unexplained postmenopausal bleeding, has abnormal glandular cells on her Pap smear, or an ultrasonogram showing a thickened endometrial stripe. Evaluation of postmenopausal bleeding or increased risk of endometrial cancer by US is a noninvasive alternative. Karlsson and colleagues[87] performed a prospective trial of transvaginal US evaluation in 1168 women with postmenopausal bleeding scheduled for D&C. These investigators found that for a US cut-off of 5 mm, no women with a stripe below 5 mm had endometrial cancer. If a postmenopausal woman has an endometrial stripe of 5 mm or greater, then her risk of endometrial cancer is found to be 31%.[88] The 5-mm threshold is only accurate in women who are postmenopausal and not using hormone replacement therapy. The use of US as a noninvasive test for evaluation of postmenopausal women is attractive because it is relatively painless and readily available. A meta-analysis has shown that the 5-mm threshold is 96% sensitive

---

Box 1
Carcinoma of the endometrium

Stage I: Tumor confined to the corpus uteri

    IA: No or less than half myometrial invasion

    IB: Invasion equal to or more than half of the myometrium

Stage II: Tumor invades cervical stroma, but does not extend beyond the uterus

Stage III: Local and/or regional spread of the tumor

    IIIA: Tumor invades the serosa of the corpus uteri and/or adnexae

    IIIB: Vaginal and/or parametrial involvement

    IIIC: Metastases to pelvic and/or para-aortic lymph nodes

        IIIC1: Positive pelvic nodes

        IIIC2: Positive para-aortic lymph nodes with or without positive pelvic lymph nodes

Stage IV: Tumor invades bladder and/or bowel mucosa, and/or distant metastases

    IVA: Tumor invasion of bladder and/or bowel mucosa

    IVB: Distant metastases, including intra-abdominal metastases and/or inguinal lymph nodes

Note: Endocervical glandular involvement only should be considered as Stage I and no longer as Stage II. Positive cytology has to be reported separately without changing the stage.
From Pecorelli S. Revised FIGO staging for carcinoma of the vulva, cervix, and endometrium. Int J Gynaecol Obstet 2009;105(2):103–4; with permission.

for detecting cancer, but has a 4% false-negative rate and a 50% false-positive rate.[89] The value of this noninvasive evaluation is in ruling out endometrial cancer without performing a biopsy. Ultimately, if the woman has a thickened stripe, then an endometrial biopsy or D&C is indicated before definitive surgery with hysterectomy.

For women diagnosed with endometrial cancer, the routine pretreatment assessment includes a thorough physical examination, laboratory studies, and a chest radiograph. Routine CT or MR imaging are not useful unless the patient is suspected of having metastatic disease.

Pretreatment or Preoperative Evaluation

The risks of lymph node staging in endometrial cancer, combined with the lack of surgical expertise and no proven benefit, invite the use of a noninvasive test that predicts metastatic disease. To date, studies of CT, MR imaging, and FDG imaging have failed to show significant benefit from the use of these modalities in the preoperative evaluation of women scheduled to undergo hysterectomy for endometrial cancer. CT and MR imaging detection of lymph node metastases are based on size, with a short-axis diameter of greater than either 8 or 10 mm as a common threshold for identifying nodal disease. The morphologic techniques have a relatively low sensitivity for detecting nodal metastases in endometrial cancer, ranging from 18% to 66%.[90–94] When endometrial cancer spreads outside the uterus, the most common patterns of spread are lymphatic to the pelvic and/or PALN, within the peritoneal cavity (most commonly with papillary serous histology), and hematogenous spread to lung, bones, or vagina. Pelvic lymph nodes are clearly the most common of the sites of metastases at the time of initial diagnosis, with most of the other sites being occult and presenting as sites of recurrence. The role of preoperative imaging is to identify patients with metastatic disease that require either more extensive surgery or a systemic therapy approach, such as chemotherapy.

The most common site of metastases at the time of diagnosis is to the regional lymph nodes; this is often micrometastatic disease for which FDG-PET/CT has a low sensitivity. In a study of 30 patients, Suzuki and colleagues[95] assessed 30 women with endometrial cancer and found that preoperative PET failed to detect the 5 cases of positive lymph node involvement when the size was 0.6 cm or less. PET was more sensitive than either CT or MR imaging for identifying other extranodal metastatic disease. The sensitivity of PET for detection of metastatic lesions was superior (83.3%) to that of CT/MR imaging (66.7%). Kitajima and colleagues[96] also investigated the accuracy of PET/CT in detecting nodal metastasis in 40 women with endometrial cancer.[95] Their study objective "was to evaluate the accuracy of integrated PET and CT (PET/CT) using ^{18}F-FDG in detecting pelvic and PALN metastasis in patients with endometrial cancer, using surgical and histopathologic findings as the reference standard." Ten of the 40 women in their study had positive lymph nodes, with this high percentage suggesting that they included a relatively high-risk population. The investigators also found a higher sensitivity for detecting lymph node metastases as the size of the involved node increased. With 60 total positive nodes found in these 10 node-positive women, the sensitivity for detecting metastatic lesions 4 mm or less in diameter was 16.7% (4/24); it was 66.7% (14/21) for lesions between 5 and 9 mm; and 93.3% (14/15) for lesions 10 mm or larger.

Because all these women require a surgical procedure unless extensive metastatic disease is present, there is no apparent benefit to the addition of preoperative staging with CT or PET scan. This finding is not surprising, given the recent cooperative group trials showing no survival benefit to systematic pelvic lymphadenectomy, which is likely more sensitive than any imaging technique. In the future, a randomized study of PET/CT imaging as compared with surgical staging and with no extended staging in a high-risk patient population would be useful in further defining the best patient management.

Treatment

The typical treatment approach for a woman with endometrial cancer is to perform a total hysterectomy and bilateral salpingo-oophorectomy, with or without lymph node dissection. This procedure can be performed by laparotomy or by using minimally invasive surgery with laparoscopy alone or with robotic assistance. The GOG Lap 2 trial showed no significant difference in survival for women treated with laparotomy versus minimally invasive surgery. The laparoscopy arm of this study had fewer moderate and severe postoperative complications and shorter length of stay.[97] Surgical assessment of the pelvic and PALNs has been the reference standard for evaluating the extent of disease in endometrial cancer since the adoption of the 1988 version of FIGO staging. Despite the decision by FIGO to include complete surgical staging with lymph node dissection, many surgeons perform only selective lymph node dissection or removal, based on prognostic factors and intraoperative findings. The risks of lymph node dissection include the acute concerns of bleeding, prolonged operative time, increased risk of thromboembolic disease, and the delayed risk of lymphedema and lymphocyst. A recent phase 3 randomized clinical trial evaluated the survival benefits of systematic pelvic lymphadenectomy for women with intermediate or high-risk early-stage endometrial cancer, defined as FIGO (1988) stage IA or B, and high-risk histology, or FIGO Stage IC/IIA. The study took place in 85 centers in 4 different countries, and included 1408 women.[98] This ASTEC (A Study of the Treatment of Endometrial Cancer) study showed no progression-free or overall survival benefit for women who underwent complete surgical staging with systematic lymphadenectomy.[98] The 5-year overall survival was 81% in the standard surgery group and 80% in the lymphadenectomy group. Critics of the study express concern that women with surgically positive pelvic lymph nodes were still randomized to receive or not receive pelvic radiotherapy. Lymphadenectomy is considered by many to be the gold standard for assessing regional metastasis, but the fact that a randomized trial showed no survival benefit suggests otherwise. Either the sensitivity of this assessment of regional metastases is too low or the results do not affect survival because they herald distant metastatic disease.

Posttreatment Surveillance

The use of an expensive surveillance tool such as FDG-PET/CT to detect recurrent disease that is rarely cured is difficult to justify. In surgical stage I endometrial cancer, the 5-year disease-free survival exceeds 90% and therefore many repeat studies would be required to detect an unlikely recurrence. The most common site of recurrence is the vagina, which can be detected clinically but may be obscured on PET/CT by the adjacent contrast within the bladder. The use of FDG imaging for recurrence surveillance was studied by Saga and colleagues[99] in a retrospective evaluation of 21 women treated surgically for endometrial cancer. FDG imaging was found to improve "diagnostic accuracy," with a sensitivity of 100%, a specificity of 88%, and an accuracy of 93%, when compared with CT or MR imaging. In an earlier publication, Belhocine and colleagues[25] studied 34 women in posttreatment surveillance, evaluating the accurate localization of suspected recurrence and detection of occult or asymptomatic recurrence, and reported a sensitivity of 96%, specificity of 78%, and accuracy of 90%. More recently, Park and colleagues[100] reported on 88 women who underwent PET/CT as posttreatment surveillance. In this study, 66 women were asymptomatic and without evidence of disease. The investigators found that treatment was changed in 22% of patients by introducing PET or PET/CT into their posttreatment surveillance. Furthermore, they note that PET/CT is highly effective in discriminating true from suspected recurrence. These high percentages imply that Park and colleagues were monitoring a high-risk patient population in this retrospective evaluation.

The routine use of FDG imaging as posttreatment surveillance has not been studied in a randomized trial and is unlikely to be cost effective. Recurrence of endometrial cancer is relatively uncommon, and timing of the diagnosis rarely affects the likelihood of salvage. The use of PET/CT may be useful, however, in treatment planning for women found to have recurrent disease.

Recurrent Endometrial Cancer

The common sites of endometrial cancer recurrence are the vagina, pelvic and PALNs, the peritoneal cavity, and lungs. Other sites of hematogenous spread, such as bone, liver, and brain, can occur but are uncommon. Vaginal recurrence of this cancer is the most common site, occurring in approximately 7% of cases. It is detected by the occurrence of bleeding and is readily apparent on vaginal examination. Vaginal recurrence can be successfully treated in 50% to 75% of cases. Other sites of recurrence, with the exception of isolated pelvic lymph nodes, are rarely salvaged. Detection of other sites of metastases generally requires imaging with CT, MR imaging, or PET/CT. Routine surveillance imaging has not proved to be effective, and likely will not be until a curative treatment for this recurrent metastatic disease is found.

FDG imaging has been shown to play an important role in the decision-making process for women with known recurrent endometrial cancer. For women with an isolated site of recurrence, surgery and/or radiotherapy may be either curative or provide effective palliation, but with multifocal recurrent disease, only palliative chemotherapy is indicated. Kitajima and colleagues[101] studied PET versus CT performance in 90 women with recurrent endometrial or cervical cancer, and found that PET improved the sensitivity and specificity for assessing the extent of disease when compared with CT. These investigators also noted that in 42% of patients, PET results led to a change of management.

Research Concepts Using Other Tracers

Studies using ^{18}F-17β-estradiol (FES) and FDG-PET have been reported in the literature by Yoshida and colleagues.[102,103] These investigators found that FES-PET is more useful in monitoring hormone therapy, especially in endometrial hyperplasia, than FDG-PET. This differential monitoring of PET signals certainly could provide valuable insights into the management of recurrent disease or fertility-sparing interventions where hormone receptor status could inform the decision to treat a woman with progestin or antiestrogen therapy rather than chemotherapy. These treatment decision strategies, however, are only theoretical and have not yet been investigated.

Endometrial cancer is a common malignancy that usually has a good prognosis. Given the favorable outcomes generally seen, there is no apparent benefit to extensive surgical or radiologic staging of these women. The utility of FDG-PET/CT is confined to clarifying the extent and location of recurrent disease, thus assisting in the individualization of salvage therapy decisions.

SUMMARY

The experience of recent years has shown that intensive teamwork yields the best results in treating gynecologic cancer patients. The team is composed of several key participants. The imaging department uses state-of-the-art technologies and accumulated experience to reach the most accurate diagnosis. The skilled physician uses innovative tools and minimally invasive procedures to achieve impressive surgical results. The modern pathologist accurately characterizes the tumor. The oncologist aptly provides the appropriate treatment according to the type and location of the tumor, combining radiation, chemotherapy, and various biologic substances.

To overcome the limitation of traditional diagnostic modalities, a combination of anatomic and metabolic imaging has been implanted in clinical practice over the last decade. This combination enhances the clinician's ability to make critical decisions in treating difficult scenarios in various gynecologic cancer patients. Further research is needed to evaluate the efficacy of PET/CT as the diagnostic modality of choice in daily clinical practice.

REFERENCES

1. Ellenson LH, Wu TC. Focus on endometrial and cervical cancer. Cancer Cell 2004;5(6):533–8.
2. Walboomers JM, Jacobs MV, Manos MM, et al. Human papillomavirus is a necessary cause of invasive cervical cancer worldwide. J Pathol 1999; 189(1):12–9.
3. Markowitz LE, Dunne EF, Saraiya M, et al. Quadrivalent human papillomavirus vaccine: recommendations of the advisory committee on immunization practices (ACIP). MMWR Recomm Rep 2007;56(RR-2):1–24.
4. Lagasse LD, Creasman WT, Shingleton HM, et al. Results and complications of operative staging in cervical cancer: experience of the Gynecologic Oncology Group. Gynecol Oncol 1980;9(1):90–8.
5. Peters WA 3rd, Liu PY, Barrett RJ 2nd, et al. Concurrent chemotherapy and pelvic radiation therapy compared with pelvic radiation therapy alone as adjuvant therapy after radical surgery in high-risk early-stage cancer of the cervix. J Clin Oncol 2000;18(8):1606–13.
6. Rose PG, Bundy BN, Watkins EB, et al. Concurrent cisplatin-based radiotherapy and chemotherapy for locally advanced cervical cancer. N Engl J Med 1999; 340(15):1144–53.
7. Sedlis A, Bundy BN, Rotman MZ, et al. A randomized trial of pelvic radiation therapy versus no further therapy in selected patients with stage IB carcinoma of the cervix after radical hysterectomy and pelvic lymphadenectomy: a Gynecologic Oncology Group Study. Gynecol Oncol 1999;73(2):177–83.
8. Grigsby PW, Siegel BA, Dehdashti F. Lymph node staging by positron emission tomography in patients with carcinoma of the cervix. J Clin Oncol 2001;19(17): 3745–9.
9. Burnett AF, Roman LD, O'Meara AT, et al. Radical vaginal trachelectomy and pelvic lymphadenectomy for preservation of fertility in early cervical carcinoma. Gynecol Oncol 2003;88(3):419–23.
10. Long HJ 3rd, Bundy BN, Grendys EC Jr, et al. Randomized phase III trial of cisplatin with or without topotecan in carcinoma of the uterine cervix: a Gynecologic Oncology Group Study. J Clin Oncol 2005;23(21):4626–33.
11. Whitcomb BP. Gynecologic malignancies. Surg Clin North Am 2008;88(2): 301–17, vi.
12. Magne N, Chargari C, Vicenzi L, et al. New trends in the evaluation and treatment of cervix cancer: the role of FDG-PET. Cancer Treat Rev 2008;34(8): 671–81.

13. Grigsby PW. The prognostic value of PET and PET/CT in cervical cancer. Cancer Imaging 2008;8:146–55.
14. Narayan K, Hicks RJ, Jobling T, et al. A comparison of MRI and PET scanning in surgically staged loco-regionally advanced cervical cancer: potential impact on treatment. Int J Gynecol Cancer 2001;11(4):263–71.
15. Singh AK, Grigsby PW, Dehdashti F, et al. FDG-PET lymph node staging and survival of patients with FIGO stage IIIb cervical carcinoma. Int J Radiat Oncol Biol Phys 2003;56(2):489–93.
16. Yeh LS, Hung YC, Shen YY, et al. Detecting para-aortic lymph nodal metastasis by positron emission tomography of ^{18}F-fluorodeoxyglucose in advanced cervical cancer with negative magnetic resonance imaging findings. Oncol Rep 2002;9(6):1289–92.
17. Yen TC, Ng KK, Ma SY, et al. Value of dual-phase 2-fluoro-2-deoxy-D-glucose positron emission tomography in cervical cancer. J Clin Oncol 2003;21(19): 3651–8.
18. Amit A, Beck D, Lowenstein L, et al. The role of hybrid PET/CT in the evaluation of patients with cervical cancer. Gynecol Oncol 2006;100(1):65–9.
19. Grigsby PW. PET/CT imaging to guide cervical cancer therapy. Future Oncol 2009;5(7):953–8.
20. Rose PG, Adler LP, Rodriguez M, et al. Positron emission tomography for evaluating para-aortic nodal metastasis in locally advanced cervical cancer before surgical staging: a surgicopathologic study. J Clin Oncol 1999;17(1):41–5.
21. Wright JD, Dehdashti F, Herzog TJ, et al. Preoperative lymph node staging of early-stage cervical carcinoma by ^{18}F]-fluoro-2-deoxy-D-glucose-positron emission tomography. Cancer 2005;104(11):2484–91.
22. Loft A, Berthelsen AK, Roed H, et al. The diagnostic value of PET/CT scanning in patients with cervical cancer: a prospective study. Gynecol Oncol 2007;106(1): 29–34.
23. Qiu JT, Ho KC, Lai CH, et al. Supraclavicular lymph node metastases in cervical cancer. Eur J Gynaecol Oncol 2007;28(1):33–8.
24. Tsai CS, Chang TC, Lai CH, et al. Preliminary report of using FDG-PET to detect extrapelvic lesions in cervical cancer patients with enlarged pelvic lymph nodes on MRI/CT. Int J Radiat Oncol Biol Phys 2004;58(5):1506–12.
25. Belhocine T, De Barsy C, Hustinx R, et al. Usefulness of (18)F-FDG PET in the post-therapy surveillance of endometrial carcinoma. Eur J Nucl Med Mol Imaging 2002;29(9):1132–9.
26. Brooks RA, Rader JS, Dehdashti F, et al. Surveillance FDG-PET detection of asymptomatic recurrences in patients with cervical cancer. Gynecol Oncol 2009;112(1):104–9.
27. Grigsby PW, Siegel BA, Dehdashti F, et al. Posttherapy ^{18}F] fluorodeoxyglucose positron emission tomography in carcinoma of the cervix: response and outcome. J Clin Oncol 2004;22(11):2167–71.
28. Tran BN, Grigsby PW, Dehdashti F, et al. Occult supraclavicular lymph node metastasis identified by FDG-PET in patients with carcinoma of the uterine cervix. Gynecol Oncol 2003;90(3):572–6.
29. Bodurka-Bevers D, Morris M, Eifel PJ, et al. Posttherapy surveillance of women with cervical cancer: an outcomes analysis. Gynecol Oncol 2000;78(2): 187–93.
30. Chien CR, Ting LL, Hsieh CY, et al. Post-radiation Pap smear for Chinese patients with cervical cancer: a ten-year follow-up. Eur J Gynaecol Oncol 2005;26(6):619–22.

31. Shield PW, Daunter B, Wright RG. Post-irradiation cytology of cervical cancer patients. Cytopathology 1992;3(3):167–82.
32. Schwarz JK, Grigsby PW, Dehdashti F, et al. The role of ^{18}F-FDG PET in assessing therapy response in cancer of the cervix and ovaries. J Nucl Med 2009; 50(Suppl 1):64S–73S.
33. Morice P, Deyrolle C, Rey A, et al. Value of routine follow-up procedures for patients with stage I/II cervical cancer treated with combined surgery-radiation therapy. Ann Oncol 2004;15(2):218–23.
34. Permuth-Wey J, Sellers TA. Epidemiology of ovarian cancer. Methods Mol Biol 2009;472:413–37.
35. Auersperg N, Wong AS, Choi KC, et al. Ovarian surface epithelium: biology, endocrinology, and pathology. Endocr Rev 2001;22(2):255–88.
36. Riman T, Nilsson S, Persson IR. Review of epidemiological evidence for reproductive and hormonal factors in relation to the risk of epithelial ovarian malignancies. Acta Obstet Gynecol Scand 2004;83(9):783–95.
37. Edwards BK, Brown ML, Wingo PA, et al. Annual report to the nation on the status of cancer, 1975-2002, featuring population-based trends in cancer treatment. J Natl Cancer Inst 2005;97(19):1407–27.
38. Ziogas A, Gildea M, Cohen P, et al. Cancer risk estimates for family members of a population-based family registry for breast and ovarian cancer. Cancer Epidemiol Biomarkers Prev 2000;9(1):103–11.
39. Malander S, Rambech E, Kristoffersson U, et al. The contribution of the hereditary nonpolyposis colorectal cancer syndrome to the development of ovarian cancer. Gynecol Oncol 2006;101(2):238–43.
40. Siskind V, Green A, Bain C, et al. Beyond ovulation: oral contraceptives and epithelial ovarian cancer. Epidemiology 2000;11(2):106–10.
41. Schutter EM, Kenemans P, Sohn C, et al. Diagnostic value of pelvic examination, ultrasound, and serum CA 125 in postmenopausal women with a pelvic mass. An international multicenter study. Cancer 1994;74(4):1398–406.
42. Schutter EM, Sohn C, Kristen P, et al. Estimation of probability of malignancy using a logistic model combining physical examination, ultrasound, serum CA 125, and serum CA 72-4 in postmenopausal women with a pelvic mass: an international multicenter study. Gynecol Oncol 1998;69(1):56–63.
43. Burghardt E, Lahousen M, Stettner H. The significance of pelvic and para-aortic lymphadenectomy in the operative treatment of ovarian cancer. Baillieres Clin Obstet Gynaecol 1989;3(1):157–65.
44. Burghardt E, Pickel H, Lahousen M, et al. Pelvic lymphadenectomy in operative treatment of ovarian cancer. Am J Obstet Gynecol 1986;155(2):315–9.
45. Dauplat J, Hacker NF, Nieberg RK, et al. Distant metastases in epithelial ovarian carcinoma. Cancer 1987;60(7):1561–6.
46. Julian CG, Goss J, Blanchard K, et al. Biologic behavior of primary ovarian malignancy. Obstet Gynecol 1974;44(6):873–84.
47. Brooks SE. Preoperative evaluation of patients with suspected ovarian cancer. Gynecol Oncol 1994;55(3 Pt 2):S80–90.
48. Curtin JP. Management of the adnexal mass. Gynecol Oncol 1994;55(3 Pt 2): S42–6.
49. Ind TE, Granowska M, Britton KE, et al. Peroperative radioimmunodetection of ovarian carcinoma using a hand-held gamma detection probe. Br J Cancer 1994;70(6):1263–6.
50. Kinkel K, Hricak H, Lu Y, et al. US characterization of ovarian masses: a meta-analysis. Radiology 2000;217(3):803–11.

51. Hewitt MJ, Anderson K, Hall GD, et al. Women with peritoneal carcinomatosis of unknown origin: Efficacy of image-guided biopsy to determine site-specific diagnosis. BJOG 2007;114(1):46–50.
52. Goff BA, Matthews BJ, Larson EH, et al. Predictors of comprehensive surgical treatment in patients with ovarian cancer. Cancer 2007;109(10):2031–42.
53. Le T, Adolph A, Krepart GV, et al. The benefits of comprehensive surgical staging in the management of early-stage epithelial ovarian carcinoma. Gynecol Oncol 2002;85(2):351–5.
54. Eisenkop SM. Commenting on centralizing surgery for gynecologic oncology: a strategy assuring better quality treatment? (89:4-8) by Karsten Munstedt, et al. Gynecol Oncol 2004;94(2):605–6 [author reply: 606–7].
55. Munstedt K, von Georgi R, Misselwitz B, et al. Centralizing surgery for gynecologic oncology—a strategy assuring better quality treatment? Gynecol Oncol 2003;89(1):4–8.
56. Boente MP, Chi DS, Hoskins WJ. The role of surgery in the management of ovarian cancer: primary and interval cytoreductive surgery. Semin Oncol 1998;25(3):326–34.
57. Chi DS, Eisenhauer EL, Lang J, et al. What is the optimal goal of primary cytoreductive surgery for bulky stage IIIC epithelial ovarian carcinoma (EOC)? Gynecol Oncol 2006;103(2):559–64.
58. Eisenkop SM, Spirtos NM, Lin WC. "Optimal" cytoreduction for advanced epithelial ovarian cancer: a commentary. Gynecol Oncol 2006;103(1):329–35.
59. Winter WE 3rd, Maxwell GL, Tian C, et al. Tumor residual after surgical cytoreduction in prediction of clinical outcome in stage IV epithelial ovarian cancer: a Gynecologic Oncology Group study. J Clin Oncol 2008;26(1):83–9.
60. Eisenhauer EL, Abu-Rustum NR, Sonoda Y, et al. The effect of maximal surgical cytoreduction on sensitivity to platinum-taxane chemotherapy and subsequent survival in patients with advanced ovarian cancer. Gynecol Oncol 2008; 108(2):276–81.
61. Redman CW, Warwick J, Luesley DM, et al. Intervention debulking surgery in advanced epithelial ovarian cancer. Br J Obstet Gynaecol 1994;101(2): 142–6.
62. Aletti GD, Gostout BS, Podratz KC, et al. Ovarian cancer surgical resectability: relative impact of disease, patient status, and surgeon. Gynecol Oncol 2006; 100(1):33–7.
63. van der Burg ME, van Lent M, Buyse M, et al. The effect of debulking surgery after induction chemotherapy on the prognosis in advanced epithelial ovarian cancer. Gynecological Cancer Cooperative Group of the European Organization for Research and Treatment of Cancer. N Engl J Med 1995; 332:629–34.
64. Rose PG, Nerenstone S, Brady MF, et al. Secondary surgical cytoreduction for advanced ovarian carcinoma. N Engl J Med 2004;351(24):2489–97.
65. Wenzel L, Huang HQ, Monk BJ, et al. Quality-of-life comparisons in a randomized trial of interval secondary cytoreduction in advanced ovarian carcinoma: a Gynecologic Oncology Group study. J Clin Oncol 2005;23(24):5605–12.
66. Ozols RF, Bundy BN, Greer BE, et al. Phase III trial of carboplatin and paclitaxel compared with cisplatin and paclitaxel in patients with optimally resected stage III ovarian cancer: a Gynecologic Oncology Group study. J Clin Oncol 2003; 21(17):3194–200.
67. Greimel ER, Bjelic-Radisic V, Pfisterer J, et al. Randomized study of the Arbeitsgemeinschaft Gynaekologische Onkologie Ovarian Cancer Study Group

comparing quality of life in patients with ovarian cancer treated with cisplatin/paclitaxel versus carboplatin/paclitaxel. J Clin Oncol 2006;24(4):579–86.

68. Einzig AI, Wiernik PH, Sasloff J, et al. Phase II study and long-term follow-up of patients treated with taxol for advanced ovarian adenocarcinoma. J Clin Oncol 1992;10(11):1748–53.

69. Heintz AP, Odicino F, Maisonneuve P, et al. Carcinoma of the ovary. FIGO 6th annual report on the results of treatment in gynecological cancer. Int J Gynaecol Obstet 2006;95(Suppl 1):S161–92.

70. Berek JS, Trope C, Vergote I. Surgery during chemotherapy and at relapse of ovarian cancer. Ann Oncol 1999;10(Suppl 1):3–7.

71. McGuire WP, Hoskins WJ, Brady MF, et al. Cyclophosphamide and cisplatin compared with paclitaxel and cisplatin in patients with stage III and stage IV ovarian cancer. N Engl J Med 1996;334(1):1–6.

72. Risum S, Hogdall C, Loft A, et al. Does the use of diagnostic PET/CT cause stage migration in patients with primary advanced ovarian cancer? Gynecol Oncol 2010;116(3):395–8.

73. Risum S, Hogdall C, Loft A, et al. The diagnostic value of PET/CT for primary ovarian cancer—a prospective study. Gynecol Oncol 2007;105(1):145–9.

74. Gu P, Pan LL, Wu SQ, et al. CA 125, PET alone, PET-CT, CT and MRI in diagnosing recurrent ovarian carcinoma: a systematic review and meta-analysis. Eur J Radiol 2009;71(1):164–74.

75. Moore RG, MacLaughlan S, Bast RC Jr. Current state of biomarker development for clinical application in epithelial ovarian cancer. Gynecol Oncol 2010;116(2):240–5.

76. Agress H Jr, Cooper BZ. Detection of clinically unexpected malignant and premalignant tumors with whole-body FDG PET: histopathologic comparison. Radiology 2004;230(2):417–22.

77. Milam RA, Milam MR, Iyer RB. Detection of early-stage ovarian cancer by FDG-PET-CT in a patient with BRCA2-positive breast cancer. J Clin Oncol 2007;25(35):5657–8.

78. Barnholtz-Sloan JS, Schwartz AG, Qureshi F, et al. Ovarian cancer: changes in patterns at diagnosis and relative survival over the last three decades. Am J Obstet Gynecol 2003;189(4):1120–7.

79. Tailor A, Bourne TH, Campbell S, et al. Results from an ultrasound-based familial ovarian cancer screening clinic: a 10-year observational study. Ultrasound Obstet Gynecol 2003;21(4):378–85.

80. Karlan BY, Baldwin RL, Lopez-Luevanos E, et al. Peritoneal serous papillary carcinoma, a phenotypic variant of familial ovarian cancer: implications for ovarian cancer screening. Am J Obstet Gynecol 1999;180(4):917–28.

81. Olivier RI, Lubsen-Brandsma MA, Verhoef S, et al. CA125 and transvaginal ultrasound monitoring in high-risk women cannot prevent the diagnosis of advanced ovarian cancer. Gynecol Oncol 2006;100(1):20–6.

82. Gadducci A, Cosio S. Surveillance of patients after initial treatment of ovarian cancer. Crit Rev Oncol Hematol 2009;71(1):43–52.

83. Jung DC, Kang S, Kim MJ, et al. Multidetector CT predictors of incomplete resection in primary cytoreduction of patients with advanced ovarian cancer. Eur Radiol 2010;20(1):100–7.

84. Gadducci A, Cosio S, Zola P, et al. Surveillance procedures for patients treated for epithelial ovarian cancer: a review of the literature. Int J Gynecol Cancer 2007;17(1):21–31.

85. Parkin DM, Bray F, Ferlay J, et al. Global cancer statistics, 2002. CA Cancer J Clin 2005;55(2):74–108.

86. Schink JC, Rademaker AW, Miller DS, et al. Tumor size in endometrial cancer. Cancer 1991;67(11):2791–4.

87. Karlsson B, Granberg S, Wikland M, et al. Transvaginal ultrasonography of the endometrium in women with postmenopausal bleeding—a Nordic multicenter study. Am J Obstet Gynecol 1995;172(5):1488–94.

88. Gupta JK, Chien PF, Voit D, et al. Ultrasonographic endometrial thickness for diagnosing endometrial pathology in women with postmenopausal bleeding: a meta-analysis. Acta Obstet Gynecol Scand 2002;81(9):799–816.

89. Tabor A, Watt HC, Wald NJ. Endometrial thickness as a test for endometrial cancer in women with postmenopausal vaginal bleeding. Obstet Gynecol 2002;99(4):663–70.

90. Hricak H, Rubinstein LV, Gherman GM, et al. MR imaging evaluation of endometrial carcinoma results of an NCI cooperative study. Radiology 1991;179(3):829–32.

91. Connor JP, Andrews JI, Anderson B, et al. Computed tomography in endometrial carcinoma. Obstet Gynecol 2000;95(5):692–6.

92. Manfredi R, Mirk P, Maresca G, et al. Local-regional staging of endometrial carcinoma: role of MR imaging in surgical planning. Radiology 2004;231(2):372–8.

93. Rockall AG, Sohaib SA, Harisinghani MG, et al. Diagnostic performance of nanoparticle-enhanced magnetic resonance imaging in the diagnosis of lymph node metastases in patients with endometrial and cervical cancer. J Clin Oncol 2005;23(12):2813–21.

94. Sugiyama T, Nishida T, Ushijima K, et al. Detection of lymph node metastasis in ovarian carcinoma and uterine corpus carcinoma by preoperative computerized tomography or magnetic resonance imaging. J Obstet Gynaecol (Tokyo 1995) 1995;21(6):551–6.

95. Suzuki R, Miyagi E, Takahashi N, et al. Validity of positron emission tomography using fluoro-2-deoxyglucose for the preoperative evaluation of endometrial cancer. Int J Gynecol Cancer 2007;17(4):890–6.

96. Kitajima K, Murakami K, Yamasaki E, et al. Accuracy of ^{18}F-FDG PET/CT in detecting pelvic and paraaortic lymph node metastasis in patients with endometrial cancer. Am J Roentgenol 2008;190(6):1652–8.

97. Walker JL, Piedmonte MR, Spirtos NM, et al. Laparoscopy compared with laparotomy for comprehensive surgical staging of uterine cancer: Gynecologic Oncology Group Study LAP2. J Clin Oncol 2009;27(32):5331–6.

98. ASTEC study group, Kitchener H, Swart AM, et al. Efficacy of systematic pelvic lymphadenectomy in endometrial cancer (MRC ASTEC trial): a randomised study. Lancet 2009;373(9658):125–36.

99. Saga T, Higashi T, Ishimori T, et al. Clinical value of FDG-PET in the follow up of post-operative patients with endometrial cancer. Ann Nucl Med 2003;17(3):197–203.

100. Park JY, Kim EN, Kim DY, et al. Clinical impact of positron emission tomography or positron emission tomography/computed tomography in the posttherapy surveillance of endometrial carcinoma: evaluation of 88 patients. Int J Gynecol Cancer 2008;18(6):1332–8.

101. Kitajima K, Murakami K, Yamasaki E, et al. Performance of integrated FDG-PET/contrast-enhanced CT in the diagnosis of recurrent uterine cancer: comparison with PET and enhanced CT. Eur J Nucl Med Mol Imaging 2009;36(3):362–72.

102. Yoshida Y, Kurokawa T, Sawamura Y, et al. The positron emission tomography with F18 17beta-estradiol has the potential to benefit diagnosis and treatment of endometrial cancer. Gynecol Oncol 2007;104(3):764–6.
103. Pecorelli S. Revised FIGO staging for carcinoma of the vulva, cervix, and endometrium. Int J Gynaecol Obstet 2009;105(2):103–4.

Pelvic Floor Imaging

Cecile A. Unger, MD[a], Milena M. Weinstein, MD[b],*,
Dolores H. Pretorius, MD[c]

KEYWORDS

- Pelvic floor disorders • Pelvic floor imaging
- Pelvic floor ultrasound • Transperineal ultrasound

Pelvic floor disorders including urinary incontinence, pelvic organ prolapse, and anal incontinence have high prevalence in women of all ages,[1] can significantly decrease quality of life, and produce an economic effect. Proper evaluation of pelvic floor muscle function, strength, and integrity is an important component of diagnosis and treatment of pelvic floor disorders. In addition, the pelvic floor muscle training used to change the structural support and strength of muscle contraction requires clinicians to be able to conduct high-quality measurements of pelvic floor muscle function and strength. Studies have shown that up to one-third of women do not know how to contract their pelvic floor muscles correctly.[2] Therefore, it is also important to be able to assess pelvic muscle function and strength to document a patient's progress during interventions designed to improve their strength.[3] Approximately 1 in 10 women undergo surgery for pelvic organ prolapse by the time they reach the age of 70 years.[4] In addition, urinary incontinence often coexists with pelvic organ prolapse.[1] Urinary incontinence is defined by the International Continence Society as a complaint of any involuntary leakage of urine.[5] The most common type of incontinence is involuntary leaking in response to increased intra-abdominal pressures during exertion, cough, or sneeze. This type of incontinence is called stress urinary incontinence.[6] Urinary incontinence is more common in women than it is in men, and it affects women of all ages. The prevalence ranges from 9% to 72%, with an incidence that rises steeply with age.[7] Several studies have documented the effects that urinary incontinence have on quality of life; it is a debilitating disorder that affects women socially and physically.[6] The International Consultation on Incontinence defines anal incontinence as the involuntary loss of gas, liquid, or stool that causes a social or hygienic

Funding: None.
The authors have nothing to disclose.
A version of this article was previously published in *Ultrasound Clinics* 5:2.
[a] Department of Vincent Obstetrics and Gynecology, Massachusetts General Hospital, 55 Fruit Street, FND 5, Boston, MA 02114, USA
[b] Division of Female Pelvic Medicine and Reconstructive Surgery, Department of Vincent Obstetrics and Gynecology, Massachusetts General Hospital, 55 Fruit Street, FND 5, Boston, MA 02114, USA
[c] Department of Radiology, University of California San Diego, San Diego, CA, USA
* Corresponding author.
E-mail address: mweinstein2@partners.org

Obstet Gynecol Clin N Am 38 (2011) 23–43
doi:10.1016/j.ogc.2011.02.002
0889-8545/11/$ – see front matter © 2011 Elsevier Inc. All rights reserved.

problem.[8] The prevalence of anal incontinence has been documented in several studies to range from 20% to 54%.[9,10] The underlying cause of this type of incontinence is often related to anal sphincter defects following vaginal deliveries.[11] Because these disorders are so prevalent and severely affect a woman's quality of life, it is important to understand normal pelvic anatomy and function to treat pelvic floor disorders appropriately.[12]

PELVIC FLOOR ANATOMY AND FUNCTION

The deep muscles of the pelvic floor are often referred to as the levator ani or the pelvic diaphragm. The muscles that comprise the levator ani include the pubococcygeus, puborectalis, and iliococcygeus. These muscles span the space between the obturator internus muscle laterally, the pubis symphysis anteriorly, and the coccyx posteriorly. The superficial muscles of the pelvic floor make up the urogenital diaphragm and include the ischiocavernosus, bulbospongiosus, and the transverses perinea superficialis (**Fig. 1**). These pelvic floor muscles are encased in fascia that is continuous with the endopelvic fascia, which surrounds the pelvic viscera and also contributes to pelvic support.[3] The levator hiatus is a funnel-shaped cleft in the muscles of the levator ani from which exit the urethra, vagina, and anal canal.[13] The puborectalis is the most inferior muscle of the pelvic floor and is composed of 2 limbs attached to the 2 pubic rami anteriorly; they merge posterior to the anal canal.[14] A normal anal canal is approximately 4 cm and represents the most distal portion of the gastrointestinal tract. The anal verge demarcates its most distal end. The structures surrounding the anal canal are responsible for maintaining fecal continence and include the involuntary internal anal sphincter (IAS), the voluntary external anal sphincter (EAS), and the puborectalis muscle (PRM). The IAS is responsible for approximately 80% of resting anal tone and where it terminates distally represents the junction of the subcutaneous and superficial components of the EAS, which is created from the downward extension of the PRM. The rectum, which is in communication with the anal canal, contains a longitudinal

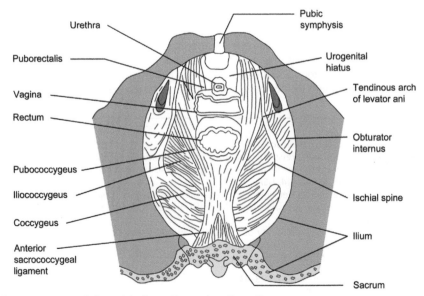

Fig. 1. Anatomy of the pelvic floor. Illustration: Rose Katz.

muscle layer that extends distally, separating the EAS and IAS, and anchors the sphincter complex to the fascia of the levator ani, as well as the pelvic side wall.[15] The perineal body separates the anus from the vagina. It is the central portion of the perineum that represents where the EAS, the bulbospongiosus, and the superficial and deep transverse perineal muscles meet. The presence of a thick perineal body is suggestive of a normal anal sphincter.[16]

The important role of the pelvic floor musculature is to perform voluntary contractions as well as involuntary, or reflex, contractions preceding or at the time of increased abdominal pressure. These types of contractions preserve fecal and urinary continence. In response to increased abdominal pressures, the superficial pelvic muscles, such as the anal and urethral sphincters, resist these pressures; and the levator ani muscles support the pelvic floor and counteract these pressures by contracting and creating a circular closing of the levator hiatus and an upward movement of the pelvic floor and perineum.[17–20] The PRM has an important role in pelvic floor support and conservation of continence. When this muscle contracts, the length of its 2 limbs is reduced, and this change lifts the anal canal anteriorly, compressing the structures within the levator hiatus against each other as well as the back of the pubic symphysis.[21] Because of their important role in urethral closure for urinary continence, these muscles are the target tissue in physical therapy for management of incontinence and other pelvic floor disorders.[22] In addition to the pelvic floor muscles, another important factor for urinary continence is the smooth and striated muscle contraction within the urethral wall, as well as the ligaments and the fascia that support the bladder and urethra in proper position during increased intra-abdominal pressure.[23] Fecal continence is maintained by the anorectal lift of the pelvic floor as well as the constricting of the anal canal. Urinary continence is preserved by the support applied to the bladder neck during pelvic floor contraction, as well as constriction of the urethral lumen.[17,18]

CONVENTIONAL IMAGING OF THE PELVIC FLOOR

Many imaging modalities have previously been used to evaluate the pelvic floor, including computed tomography, magnetic resonance (MR) imaging, and barium defecography.[24–26] These various forms of imaging have enhanced the diagnosis of many pelvic floor disorders, including pelvic organ prolapse.[12,27] Defecography uses fluoroscopy to evaluate the pelvic floor. It is an imaging modality that is appropriate for assessing pelvic organ prolapse because it uses contrast material to opacify the involved organs and it is used to evaluate their function in real time. The advantage of defecography is that it replicates the patient's symptoms, because it requires the patient to be upright during the evaluation. Organs of the anterior and posterior compartments of the pelvic floor can be examined, so that a patient can be evaluated for anterior and posterior prolapse.[25] Although defecography is useful to evaluate the interaction of rectal evacuation with the other pelvic organs and their relationship with the pelvic floor musculature, there is a significant disadvantage to defecography: it requires multiorgan opacification, which exposes patients to high-level radiation.[24,28] In addition, no studies have evaluated the reproducibility of the measurements obtained during defecography.

MR is used to evaluate the gross morphology of the pelvic floor anatomy and provides advanced soft-tissue differentiation because of its high spatial resolution. In addition, MR provides multiplanar imaging but avoids ionizing radiation and contrast material; it is also advantageous because it is not operator dependent.[25] T1-weighted images are usually taken in multiple planes. Coronal images show the structures from the anal verge to where the EAS meets the levator ani. Images can also be taken at the level of the puborectalis plane, which enables visualization of the IAS, EAS, and the levator ani, which makes this modality an excellent tool to evaluate for sphincter abnormalities and structural causes for incontinence.[25] The disadvantages of MR imaging are that it is the most expensive modality, it is time consuming, and it is not always readily available.[24,25,29] A significant disadvantage of using MR is its poor dynamic parameters in assessing pelvic organ descent during patient straining or squeezing and the need to place patients in nonphysiologic positions to look for prolapse.[25,29] Studies have shown that the prolapse parameters measured on MR correlate poorly with those seen on defecography[25] and therefore it is difficult to assess the degree of prolapse found in patients who undergo MR imaging.

ULTRASOUND IMAGING

Ultrasound has been widely used to explore pelvic floor abnormalities and dysfunction.[30–32] Real-time ultrasound can be used to look at the dynamic interaction involved in the pelvic floor as it relates to continence and pelvic organ prolapse. Studies have shown that ultrasound is superior as a clinical adjunct when compared with conventional methods, including anal manometry, electromyography, and defecography.[33] It is especially useful as a biofeedback tool for pelvic floor training.[19]

Endoanal Ultrasound

Endoanal ultrasound can be used to evaluate the anal sphincter complex to assist in the diagnosis of fecal incontinence. Many studies have shown that on ultrasound, fecal incontinence is strongly associated with anal sphincter defects; patients most often have a combined external and internal sphincter defect, or an EAS defect alone; isolated internal sphincter defects are rare.[16,34]

Endoanal ultrasound requires a high frequency transducer of 7 mHz or higher that can produce a 360° panoramic image to adequately visualize the anal sphincter complex.[35] Patients are usually placed in a prone or left lateral position because this facilitates the complete imaging of the anterior part of the sphincter complex as well as the perineum. Once the transducer is placed in the anal canal, it is rotated to the 12 o'clock position anteriorly. When the transducer is rotated in this direction, the images obtained are in the same orientation as those used for cross-sectional imaging of the entire body.[15] In this view, 4 anatomic layers can be visualized: the subepithelial layer, which is hyperechoic; the IAS, which is a hypoechoic ring with a thickness of approximately 1.35 to 2.67 mm; the longitudinal muscle, which is hyperechoic; and the EAS, which is hyperechoic and is the outermost layer, with a measured thickness of approximately 5.4 to 7.42 mm.[15,35] In the most cephalad region of the anal canal, the deep EAS is continuous with the PRM, which is a sling of mixed echogenicity that loops posteriorly around the anal canal (**Fig. 2**).[15]

Ultrasound allows for an easy visualization of the anal canal structures and thus is a perfect tool to assess the integrity of these structures.[25] Anal sphincter defects are seen as thickening and changes of echogenicity or asymmetry along the sphincter, described based on a clock face on which 12 o'clock is at the anterior position. Defects in the EAS appear hypoechoic, whereas defects in the IAS appear hyperechoic (**Fig. 3**).[15] Studies have shown good intraobserver and interobserver agreement on recognition of sphincter defects using endoanal ultrasound.[36] Results have also correlated with anorectal manometry findings in other studies; defects in the EAS are associated with lower anal squeeze pressures, whereas defects in the IAS are associated with lower resting anal pressures.[37,38] Endoanal ultrasound is considered

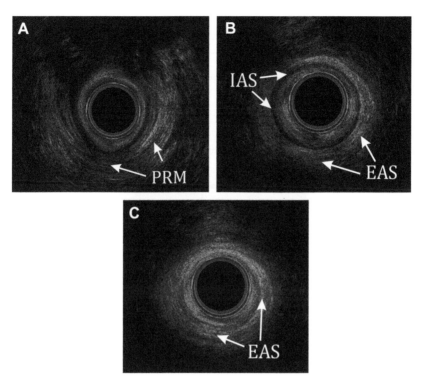

Fig. 2. Endoanal ultrasound with normal anal sphincter complex. (*A*) Proximal anal canal with puborectalis: endoanal ultrasound transducer is the round black circle in the middle, surrounded by echolucent anal mucosa and dark ring of the IAS. The IAS is surrounded posteriorly with the posterior portion of the PRM (*arrows*). (*Courtesy of* Dr Liliana Bordeianou.) (*B*) Midanal canal: the echolucent circle of the IAS (*arrows*), which is surrounded by an echogenic circle of the EAS (*arrows*). (*Courtesy of* Dr Liliana Bordeianou.) (*C*) Distal anal canal: the superficial portion of echogenic EAS (*arrows*) seen surrounding the transducer. This portion of EAS extends further distally than the IAS, which is normally not visible at the most distal extend of the anal canal. (*Courtesy of* Dr Liliana Bordeianou.)

to be a sensitive study for anal sphincter defects; with sensitivity reaching 100% in some studies. This finding has been determined by comparing ultrasound findings with surgical findings at the time of anal sphincter repair for fecal incontinence, whereas other studies have compared ultrasound findings with sphincter defects confirmed histologically.[39–41] Furthermore, studies have shown that endoanal ultrasound can be used to show resolution of sphincter defects after sphincteroplasty, which has good correlation with patients' symptoms and resolution of incontinence.[42,43] Endoanal ultrasound can also be used as a means to detect sphincter defects early, before development of incontinence symptoms. Faltin and colleagues[44] showed that the use of ultrasound in addition to a standard clinical examination immediately post partum improved the detection of anal sphincter tears. The immediate repair of these tears significantly decreased the risk of severe fecal incontinence reported 3 months to 1 year after giving birth.

Perineal body measurement has been reported to enhance the evaluation of anal sphincter defects. This measurement can be obtained by positioning the patient in the left lateral position, placing the endoanal transducer inside the rectum, and slowly

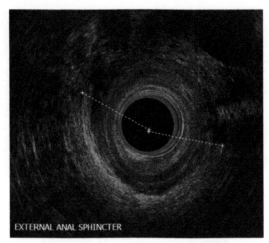

Fig. 3. Endoanal ultrasound of the midanal canal showing external and IAS defect (*shown with calipers*); the sphincter damage spans the area between 10 o'clock and 3 o'clock. (*Courtesy of* Dr Liliana Bordeianou.)

withdrawing the transducer so that the anal canal is visualized. A gloved finger is placed into the vagina and pressure is held against the posterior vaginal wall at the level of the midanal canal. The distance between the sonographic reflection of the fingertip and the inner border of the subepithelial layer is measured on a frozen ultrasound image.[16] Studies have found that thinning of the perineal body is a clinical finding among incontinent women who have anal sphincter defects. It has been shown that patients with a perineal body thickness of 10 mm or less are likely to have an anal sphincter defect 93% to 97% of the time.[16,45] Patients with a perineal body thickness of 10 to 12 mm are shown to have an indeterminate thickness of the perineal body, and anal sphincter defects can be found in approximately one-third of these patients. A perineal body thickness of greater than 12 mm was shown to be unlikely to be associated with a sphincter defect unless a patient had previously undergone reconstructive perineal surgery, at which point the risk of a defect was shown to be approximately 20%.[16]

Because the images obtained show the entire anal canal as it relates to the sphincter complex and the rest of the pelvic floor, endoanal ultrasound can be used to delineate fistulas, abscesses, and anal carcinomas.[25] Fistulas appear as hypoechoic tracts containing pockets of air that appear as focal hyperechoic areas.[15] The technique has also been used to evaluate patients with obstructed defecation, which is visualized as thickening of the sphincter muscle complex.[46] Patients with pelvic organ prolapse and urinary incontinence can also be evaluated with endoanal ultrasound. Patients with urinary incontinence have concomitant anal sphincter defects noted on endoanal ultrasound 52% of the time, and patients with other pelvic floor disorders have been shown to have additional anal sphincter defects 30% of the time.[34] These findings have been replicated in other studies as well, proving that there is a spectrum of pelvic floor disorders, with extensive overlap amongst the defects that can be seen on ultrasound.[47]

Endoanal ultrasound has also been used as biofeedback during pelvic floor exercises that are used to strengthen pelvic floor muscles for patients with prolapse and incontinence symptoms. No studies have shown that ultrasound using a transducer in the anal canal is better feedback than digital examination or anal manometry.[48] However, there is evidence that certain measurements can be obtained only with ultrasound and these measurements have better correlations with clinical outcomes than digital examination and manometry. The 2 measurements that have been studied are isotonic fatigue time and isometric fatigue contraction during pelvic floor squeezing. Pelvic floor training seems to improve these measures, which have been shown to correlate directly with a patient's improvement in quality of life and improvement in fecal continence symptoms. Endoanal ultrasound may not have any additional benefit during a physical therapy session in regards to biofeedback, compared with conventional methods of feedback; however, it seems that ultrasound may have an important role in determining physiologic measures, which correlate well with pelvic floor strength and improvement with training.[48]

Transperineal Ultrasound

Transperineal ultrasound was one of the first modes of ultrasound to be used to evaluate the soft tissues and viscera of the pelvic floor. An article written by Beer-Gabel and colleagues[24] describes the following technique for the use of transperineal ultrasound. The patient is positioned in the left lateral position, and acoustic gel is applied to the vagina and rectum. In other studies, patients have been placed in the dorsal supine lithotomy position.[49] The ultrasound transducer is then placed on the perineal body in the midsagittal plane to outline the pelvic floor muscles and organs. Images are obtained at rest, during maximal straining (Valsalva maneuver), and during pelvic squeeze so that real-time movement can be assessed. The transducer is then rotated 180° to visualize the anus and its surrounding structures, including the EAS and IAS. Sagittal evaluation of the anterior portion of the perineum shows the distal vagina, bladder, and urethra as well as the rectovaginal septum. These images are useful for the diagnosis of anterior vaginal wall prolapse (cystocele), posterior vaginal wall prolapse (rectocele), and for measuring the vaginal vault prolapse. Certain anatomic measurements can be taken in this view. These measurements include the perimeters of the PRM and the calculation of the anorectal angle as well as the posterior urethrovesical angle. The anorectal angle is measured where the longitudinal axis of the anal canal (designated with a line) meets the posterior border of the rectal wall. The urethrovesical angle or the urethrovesical junction is measured by creating a perpendicular line from the x-axis on the image, and following this line to the margin of the bladder base when the patient is at rest (**Fig. 4**).[50] The anorectal angle and the urethrovesical angle are measured at rest and at squeeze, which is helpful in the diagnosis of fecal incontinence, organ prolapse, and urinary incontinence.[24] In addition, this view allows for the dynamic function of the puborectalis to be measured. The puborectalis is visualized as a hyperechoic sling hugging the IAS in the transverse view and as a soft-tissue bundle in the sagittal view. The distance between the posterior margin of the symphysis pubis and posterior limit of the anorectal junction represents the perimeter of the puborectalis. The difference in length between the rest measurement and the squeeze measurement defines the dynamic activity of this muscle; the muscle usually shortens during a contraction (**Fig. 5**). When the transducer head is held in the transverse plane, oriented backward at 45°, at the level of the vaginal introitus, a different view of the anal sphincters can be captured as well. As in the longitudinal axis, the IAS appears hypoechoic, whereas the EAS appears hyperechoic.[24,49]

Transperineal ultrasound can be a useful tool. Investigators have described it as being applicable from a clinical perspective. It can be used to visualize the anal sphincter complex, which is useful in the grading of hemorrhoidal disease, evaluating the submucosal location of anal fistulas, and looking at sphincter defects. Studies have looked at the usefulness of conducting a physical examination alone after repair of a perineal injury from childbirth, versus using transperineal sonography as well to

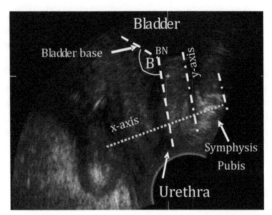

Fig. 4. The posterior urethrovesical angle measurement method with perineal ultrasound described by Schaer and colleagues.[50] The rectangular coordinate system was constructed with the y-axis at the inferior symphysis pubis and the x-axis perpendicular through the mid-symphysis pubis. The posterior urethrovesical angle (B) was measured with a line through the urethral axis and the other line through the at least one-third of the bladder base.

ensure proper sphincter repair. The digital examination is adequate to ensure proper restoration of the anatomy, which includes palpating for EAS thickness and perineal body length; however, ultrasound was determined to enhance evaluation by providing additional information on sphincter function.[51]

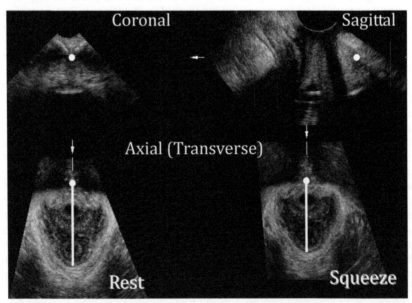

Fig. 5. Transperineal three-dimensional ultrasound of the pelvic floor hiatus: multiplanar image with coronal, sagittal, and axial (transverse) planes shown. The original volume was obtained at rest; the insert image of the axial pelvic floor hiatus is from a volume obtained during a sustained pelvic floor contraction (squeeze). Images show measures on the anterior-posterior (AP) hiatal length; the shortening of the AP length is a reflection of shortening as a result of the PRM shortening during pelvic floor contraction.

Endoanal ultrasound has been reported as one of the most reliable methods of identifying anal sphincter defects. However, images obtained by transperineal ultrasound have shown the same concentric layers and cross-sectional images as seen on endoanal ultrasound.[49] Many support the use of transperineal ultrasound for these reasons, as well as the other advantages, which include low cost, availability of equipment, and low degree of invasiveness for the patient.[49] It can also be used to visualize the contrast between the shapes of the pelvic organs at rest and during straining, which helps to diagnose posterior and anterior vaginal wall prolapse (rectocele and cystocele), enteroceles, and genital prolapse.[24] In addition, the urethrovesical junction during straining can be measured, which is useful for the diagnosis of stress urinary incontinence. Minardi and Parri[52] used transperineal ultrasound to assess the function and morphology of the urethral sphincter and detrusor muscle in the evaluation of dysfunctional voiding in patients with recurrent urinary tract infections. Via transperineal ultrasound, the urethrovesical angle, proximal pubourethral distance, and the urethral inclination were measured and calculated. The thickness of the bladder detrusor wall was measured at the bladder dome via a suprapubic ultrasound. The urethral sphincter volume was then measured with a transvaginal ultrasound transducer. They were able to show that patients who had recurrent urinary tract infections and dysfunctional voiding, shown on urodynamic testing, had higher urethral sphincter volumes and abnormal echogenicity of the urethral sphincters. In addition, they were able to use the calculated measurements of the posterior urethrovesical angle, proximal pubourethral distance, and the urethral inclination to diagnose urethral hypermobility, which was more common in patients with recurrent infections. Urodynamic testing on these patients significantly correlated with the calculated urethral sphincter volumes on ultrasound, showing the validity of these measurements. With all of this information, the investigators were able to create threshold ultrasound measurements for patients with dysfunctional voiding, and they propose that transperineal ultrasound be used as a first-line diagnostic test for evaluating patients with suspected urinary incontinence.[52]

Three-dimensional Ultrasound

Three-dimensional ultrasound has been used for the last 20 years and has been embraced by the obstetrics specialty in the last 5 years. Gynecologists are now starting to use this modality as an adjunct to study pelvic floor disorders.[53,54]

As mentioned earlier, MR imaging has been one of the modalities of choice for evaluation of the pelvic floor because it can identify the involved muscle groups, and has excellent spatial resolution. However, the major limitation of MR imaging is its failure to fully capture present-time pictures because spatial resolution is often spared as imaging time becomes faster. It is also expensive and time consuming and is less clinically convenient. As a result, the usefulness of three-dimensional ultrasound has been studied.[13,14,21,55]

Some studies have shown poor correlation between MR imaging and ultrasound, but some investigators believe that this is because previous studies did not use the same plane on ultrasound as was used on MR.[13] Another study showed that the 2 modalities correlate at rest, but there is no correlation during maximum Valsalva. This finding is likely because of the physical limitations of MR imaging. When using MR imaging, it is difficult to predict the end point during Valsalva and because MR is not performed under real time, the true plane needed to adequately evaluate pelvic floor function is not as available to the degree that it is in ultrasound.[13] In more recent studies, transperineal three-dimensional ultrasound has shown to be as effective, if not better, than MR imaging in imaging the pelvic floor.[13] This is because three-dimensional ultrasound contains cine loop capabilities, which allows for assessment of the functional anatomy of the pelvic floor with superior spatial and temporal resolution with multiple volumes of imaging obtained per second.[56] Three-dimensional ultrasound acquires volume datasets that can be used to produce single slices in any arbitrarily defined plane.[47]

The three-dimensional ultrasound technique used to evaluate the pelvic floor was described in a recent study conducted by Weinstein and colleagues.[14] The imaging is performed with subjects in the dorsal supine lithotomy position, using a transvaginal transducer placed on the midperineum, oriented in the midsagittal plane to obtain images of the anal sphincter complex. The ultrasound beam is directed in the cranial direction to visualize the pelvic floor hiatus as well as the PRM. The field of view is optimized by identifying the symphysis pubis on the left of the screen and the anal canal on the right side of the screen (**Fig. 6A**).[14] When the beam is directed in the posterior direction, the EAS and IAS are visualized. Images are captured at rest and during sustained anal sphincter and pelvic floor contraction. To visualize the anal sphincters

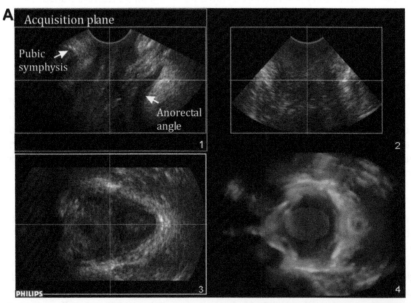

Fig. 6. (*A*) Transperineal ultrasound of the pelvic floor hiatus. Endovaginal ultrasound transducer positioned on the perineum and oriented cranially to obtain the three-dimensional volume. The acquisition plane-sagittal plane is optimized by visualizing the pubic symphysis and the anorectal angle. (*B*) Volume is rotated to orient the axial plane upright. The multiplanar of the three-dimensional transperineal volume is shown with coronal, sagittal, and axial (transverse) planes. (*C*) The dot marker is moved in the axial (transverse) plane in the area of the pubic symphysis. The pubic rami and pubic symphysis are visible in the coronal plane. The dot marker is positioned on the pubic symphysis. (*D*) In the sagittal plane the volume is rotated to align the pubic symphysis with the anorectal angle; this represents the PRM plane. The PRM is seen encircling the pelvic floor hiatus in the transverse image. (*E*) The transperineal view of the pelvic floor hiatus after completion of the volume rotation. The rendered thick slice (10 mm) allows for more detailed assessment of the hiatal structures. The pelvic floor hiatus anatomy includes a cross section of the urethra, vagina, and the anorectum. The hiatus is encircled by the PRM. The PRM can also be seen as a bundle abutting the anorectum at the anorectal angle in the sagittal plane.

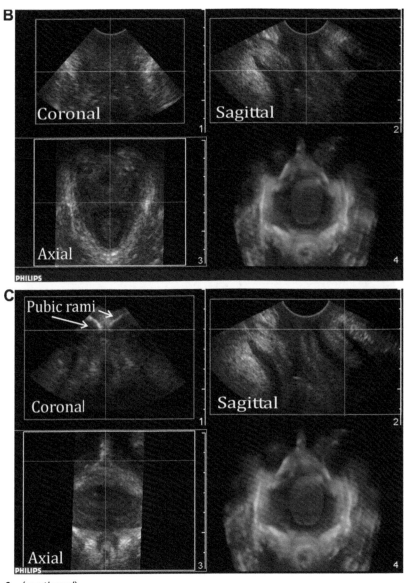

Fig. 6. (*continued*)

three-dimensionally, the sagittal images of the anal canal are rotated in the horizontal direction and the axial images that are examined are the craniocaudal length of the IAS and EAS at 1-mm distances separating each image (**Fig. 7**). The lower edge of the pubic symphysis and anorectal angles are then identified and these landmarks are used to delineate the PRM. The puborectalis plane is defined by a straight line that connects these 2 landmarks (see **Fig. 6**A–D). The puborectalis inner perimeter is defined by a curvilinear measurement along the inner border of the PRM to its insertion site on the pubic ramus. The pelvic floor hiatus inner area is defined as the area within the PRM inner perimeter enclosed anteriorly by 2 straight lines, connecting the puborectalis insertion point on the pubic rami to the inferior edge of the symphysis pubis.

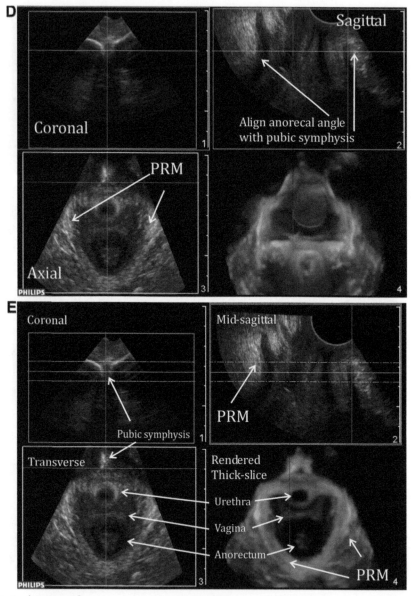

Fig. 6. (*continued*)

The pelvic floor hiatus outer area is contained within the outer border of the puborec-talis; it has the same borders as the pelvic floor hiatus inner area anteriorly. The pubor-ectalis area is a calculated measurement obtained by subtracting the pelvic floor hiatus from the outer area. This measurement represents the cross-sectional area of the puborectalis.[14] Images are captured parallel to this plane, again, at 1-mm distances separating each image. In addition, a 10-mm-thick slice is captured, which integrates the volumes of data obtained (see **Fig. 6E**). This tool is used to assess the anatomic appearance of the muscles examined for any defects, to ensure that any

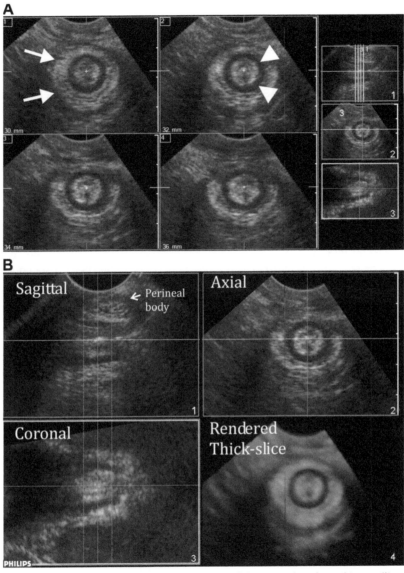

Fig. 7. (*A*) Cross-sectional (axial) multislice imaging of the normal anal canal in a nulliparous woman. The anal sphincter complex is shown at every 2-mm distance using the I-Slice function. The arrowheads mark the hypoechoic (*dark circle*) IAS; the arrows mark the hyperechoic (*white*) outer ring EAS; both sphincters are uniform and symmetric. The PRM is not seen here because the cross section is through the midportion of the sphincter complex and the PRM is a more caudal structure. (*B*) Transperineal three-dimensional ultrasound of the normal anal canal: the multiplanar of the ultrasound of the normal anal sphincter is shown with the corresponding planes: sagittal, coronal, and axial (cross-sectional). The rendered thick slice (10 mm) allows for integrated evaluation of the midanal sphincter portion. In the sagittal plane the perineal body is seen as an oval structure.

defects noted on the two-dimensional images are real and not artifact. A shift from the midline in any of the pelvic floor hiatal structures is also measured, as any defect in the puborectalis may cause asymmetry in the pelvic floor hiatus. The anterior-posterior length of the pelvic floor hiatus is also calculated. This length is described as the distance between the pubic symphysis and an anorectal angle.[14]

Three-dimensional ultrasound has been shown to be a reliable method for detecting morphologic defects in the IAS, EAS, and puborectalis.[55] These defects have been identified in studies of women after childbirth, because this population has a high incidence of PRM and anal sphincter defects related to childbirth trauma.[57] Studies have shown that the most common injury related to childbirth is an avulsion injury of the insertion of the PRM on the pubic ramus (**Fig. 8**).[58] Detecting avulsions of the PRM has a potential clinical implication in women with fecal incontinence.[58,59] Contractions of the PRM are believed to decrease the anorectal angle and increase pressure in the proximal part of the anal canal, and when the EAS contracts, there is increased pressure in the distal part of the canal.[60] On three-dimensional ultrasound, these contractions and associated measurements are well captured.[61] Three-dimensional ultrasound can also visualize anatomic defects of the individual components of the anal sphincter (**Fig. 9**). For example, the anal canal may appear asymmetric when there is a defect, and this asymmetry is more pronounced during pelvic floor contraction or squeeze. Patients with fecal incontinence are shown to have sphincter complex and PRM defects compared with nulliparous patients with no symptoms of incontinence. Women who are parous and examined with ultrasound are shown to have more defects than nulliparous women, but fewer abnormalities when compared with women who have diagnosed fecal incontinence. In addition, women noted to have an anatomically defective puborectalis have longer anterior-posterior lengths of the pelvic floor hiatus compared with controls. Other measurements that can be obtained with three-dimensional ultrasound include the muscular component of the levator hiatus (the length of the suprapubic arch subtracted from the hiatal circumference) and the muscle strain on contraction (hiatal circumference subtracted from the hiatal circumference at rest). These measurements can raise suspicion for levator injuries or defects if they are abnormal. In addition, the images can be used to look for avulsion injuries, which appear as abnormal insertion of the PRM on the inferior pubic ramus. This image is best seen during maximal contraction of the pelvic floor (**Fig. 10**).[62]

Transperineal three-dimensional ultrasound has been compared with two-dimensional endoanal ultrasound and has been shown to be a better mode of imaging

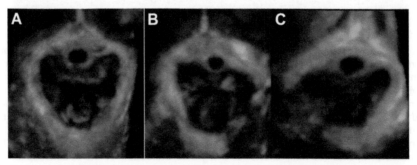

Fig. 8. An example of hiatal structure and the PRM without injury are shown (*A*). Examples of the PRM injury (*B, C*) on 10-mm-thick slice images of the PRM. The PRM injury is easily seen with asymmetry in hiatal structures. Note how urethra and vagina shift away from the midline to the side where the PRM injury is greater.

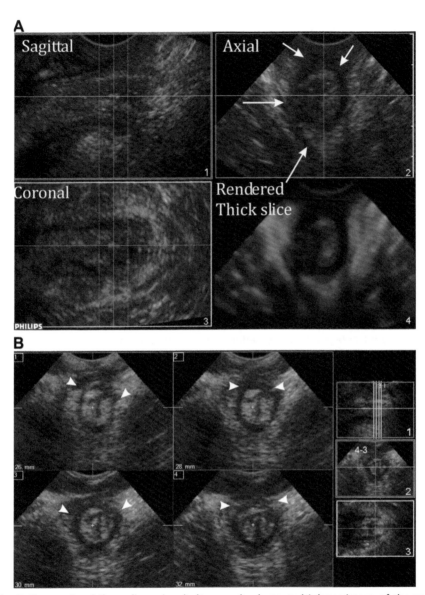

Fig. 9. Transperineal three-dimensional ultrasound volume multiplanar image of the anal sphincter complex from 2 patients with anal sphincter defect. (*A*) The anal sphincter defect is shown with arrows and affects the anterior portion of the IAS and EAS as well as the area between 7 and 9 o'clock. The rendered 10-mm-thick slice allows for enhanced assessment of the sphincter damage in the midanal canal. (*B*) The multislice image of the anal sphincter complex with 2-mm slices through the midportion of the anal canal. This example shows defect of the EAS, which also involves the IAS at the anterior aspect, between approximately 11 and 1 o'clock (*arrowheads*). The anal mucosa shows asymmetry toward the area of the EAS/IAS defect.

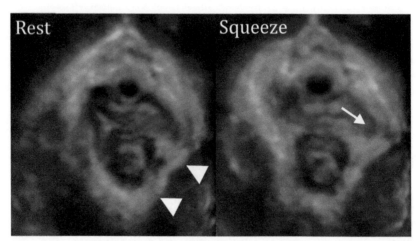

Fig. 10. Dynamic images of the pelvic floor hiatus at rest and during squeeze in the same parous woman. The injury of the PRM (*arrowheads*) is accentuated when during the pelvic floor contraction (squeeze) the pelvic floor hiatus bulges out toward the side of injury (*arrow*).

with many advantages. It allows better visualization of the entire puborectalis sling, which is not seen well on two-dimensional imaging.[21] In addition, using a cutaneous transducer is less invasive and is favored by patients, there is less operator-induced error in capturing adequate images, thin and thick slices of the ultrasound images are available, the entire pelvic hiatus can be visualized as well as any asymmetry in the hiatus or the vagina, and structures in the hiatus are well delineated compared with two-dimensional imaging. However, three-dimensional ultrasound is new technology and it is still at the preliminary stages of its clinical application in most clinical sites.

ULTRASOUND IN THE EVALUATION AND TREATMENT OF URINARY INCONTINENCE

Three-dimensional ultrasound has also been used in the assessment of patients with urinary incontinence by imaging the urethral morphology and measuring the urethra and its sphincter. Imaging has shown that women with stress urinary incontinence have urethral sphincters that are shorter, thinner, and smaller in volume.[63] There has been debate about the urinary continence mechanism, whether it is related to an extrinsic mechanism such as a sling that is located under the urethra that is pulled upward and compresses the urethra during pelvic floor contraction,[64] or whether it is related to an intrinsic mechanism such as striated sphincter that contracts down on the urethral lumen when the pelvic muscles contract.[65] With use of three-dimensional ultrasound Umek and colleagues[66] tried to elucidate the urethral continence mechanism. With use of a transrectal transducer, the morphology of the urethra was recorded and the urethral diameters, sphincter, and smooth muscle lengths as well as their thickness and volumes were measured. These investigators found that urethral diameters and sphincter thickness were smaller during pelvic floor contraction compared with pelvic floor relaxation. In addition, total urethral and sphincter volumes are smaller during contraction compared with relaxation. The smooth muscle complex of the urethra did not change in thickness or volume during contraction periods compared with relaxation periods. These investigators concluded that the urethral continence mechanism was extrinsic and occurs because of external compression by paraurethral tissues rather than intrinsic contraction of the urethral sphincter.[66]

Urethral bulking agents are used to improve continence by enhancing urethral coaptation. These agents are mostly used in urinary disorders that are attributed to intrinsic sphincter abnormalities or urethral hypermobility.[67] In 1993, Khuller and colleagues[68] imaged women using two-dimensional transperineal and transvaginal ultrasound after periurethral collagen injections. These investigators first correlated clinical symptoms of incontinence with urodynamic testing to test for improved sphincter function. They subsequently evaluated the collagen around the urethra with ultrasound and found that the parameter that was most correlated with improvement in continence was collagen intrusion into the bladder base, and not the cross-sectional area of the collagen. They concluded that increased collagen at the bladder neck improves clinical outcomes. This finding has also been replicated in other studies.[69] Studies have also reported an optimal periurethral location for bulking agents. This finding has been assessed using three-dimensional ultrasound, which is considered the best way to evaluate this parameter because it can measure the volumes of irregularly shaped structures; these measurements have been proved to be reproducible and reliable.[53] These studies have shown that the optimal periurethral location of the collagen is a circumferential or horseshoe distribution around the urethra. This type of distribution contributes to a 60% to 80% improvement in continence, whereas an asymmetric distribution is associated with a significantly smaller improvement in continence symptoms.[53,70,71] Poon and Zimmern[53] describe the use of three-dimensional ultrasound as part of their standard algorithm in managing incontinence in patients who undergo periurethral collagen injection. If a patient has no or minimal improvement after collagen injection therapy and ultrasound shows low volume retention of collagen or an asymmetric distribution, the patient is offered a repeat injection in the area of deficiency. If there is no improvement but a circumferential pattern is seen on ultrasound, the injection is considered optimal and the patient is offered an alternative treatment.

Ultrasound can also show the spatial relationship between a suburethral sling, the urethra, and the symphysis pubis at rest and on Valsalva. Urethral slings are usually made out of mesh material, which is easily visualized on ultrasound because it is echogenic. It has been shown to move variably as an arc around the posterior symphysis pubis. Movement closes the gap between the mesh and the bony structure of the pelvic, thereby compressing the urethra during increases in intra-abdominal pressure. The ability to visualize the variability in the location and the movement of the sling allows clinicians to understand why there is variability in the efficacy of the sling and to help determine if the sling needs to be adjusted.[72]

SUMMARY

In summary, pelvic floor ultrasound is a valuable adjunct in elucidation of cause, diagnosis, and treatment of pelvic floor disorders. Three-dimensional ultrasound specifically has been shown to have many advantages over conventional imaging modalities. When using three-dimensional ultrasound, scanning times are short and the technique is noninvasive; there is less user dependency when compared with two-dimensional ultrasound, which contributes to the accuracy of measurements, there is no radiation exposure involved, and it allows for the capturing of images in real time.[53] In addition, three-dimensional ultrasound has proved to be especially useful in the imaging of pelvic organ prolapse as well as the evaluation and treatment of urinary and fecal incontinence, which are disorders that many women face. Proper evaluation of pelvic floor muscle function, strength, and integrity is an important component of diagnosis and treatment of pelvic floor disorders. In addition, the pelvic floor muscle training used to change the structural support and strength of muscle contraction requires clinicians to be able to conduct high-quality measurements of pelvic floor muscle function and strength. Ultrasound has proved to be an extremely useful modality to assess the pelvic floor and its function. As practitioners become more familiar with the advantages and capabilities of ultrasound, this tool should become part of routine clinical practice in evaluation and management of pelvic floor disorders.

REFERENCES

1. Lawrence JM, Lukacz ES, Nager CW, et al. Prevalence and co-occurrence of pelvic floor disorders in community-dwelling women. Obstet Gynecol 2008; 111(3):678–85.
2. Bump RC, Hurt WG, Fantl JA, et al. Assessment of Kegel pelvic muscle exercise performance after brief verbal instruction. Am J Obstet Gynecol 1991;165(2): 322–7 [discussion: 327–9].
3. Bo K, Sherburn M. Evaluation of female pelvic-floor muscle function and strength. Phys Ther 2005;85(3):269–82.
4. Olsen AL, Smith VJ, Bergstrom JO, et al. Epidemiology of surgically managed pelvic organ prolapse and urinary incontinence. Obstet Gynecol 1997;89(4): 501–6.
5. Abrams P, Cardozo L, Fall M, et al. The standardisation of terminology of lower urinary tract function: report from the Standardisation Sub-committee of the International Continence Society. Am J Obstet Gynecol 2002;187(1):116–26.
6. Abrams P, Blaivas JG, Stanton SL, et al. Sixth report on the standardisation of terminology of lower urinary tract function. Procedures related to neurophysiological investigations: electromyography, nerve conduction studies, reflex latencies, evoked potentials and sensory testing. The International Continence Society. Br J Urol 1987;59(4):300–4.
7. Hunskaar S, Burgio K, Diokno A, et al. Epidemiology and natural history of urinary incontinence in women. Urology 2003;62(4 Suppl 1):16–23.
8. Norton CCJ, Butler U, Harari D, et al. Incontinence management. In: Abrams P, Cardozo L, Khoury S, et al, editors. Incontinence. International Consultation on Incontinence, 2001, 2002. 2nd edition. Anal incontinence, vol. 2. Plymouth (UK): Health Publications; 2002. p. 987–1043.
9. Chen GD, Hu SW, Chen YC, et al. Prevalence and correlations of anal incontinence and constipation in Taiwanese women. Neurourol Urodyn 2003;22(7):664–9.
10. Soligo M, Salvatore S, Milani R, et al. Double incontinence in urogynecologic practice: a new insight. Am J Obstet Gynecol 2003;189(2):438–43.
11. Nichols CM, Gill EJ, Nguyen T, et al. Anal sphincter injury in women with pelvic floor disorders. Obstet Gynecol 2004;104(4):690–6.
12. Shagam JY. Pelvic organ prolapse. Radiol Technol 2006;77(5):389–400 [quiz: 401–3].
13. Kruger JA, Heap SW, Murphy BA, et al. Pelvic floor function in nulliparous women using three-dimensional ultrasound and magnetic resonance imaging. Obstet Gynecol 2008;111(3):631–8.
14. Weinstein MM, Jung SA, Pretorius DH, et al. The reliability of puborectalis muscle measurements with 3-dimensional ultrasound imaging. Am J Obstet Gynecol 2007;197(1):68 e1–e6.

15. Chong AK, Hoffman B. Fecal incontinence related to pregnancy. Gastrointest Endosc Clin N Am 2006;16(1):71–81.
16. Oberwalder M, Thaler K, Baig MK, et al. Anal ultrasound and endosonographic measurement of perineal body thickness: a new evaluation for fecal incontinence in females. Surg Endosc 2004;18(4):650–4.
17. Deindl FM, Vodusek DB, Hesse U, et al. Activity patterns of pubococcygeal muscles in nulliparous continent women. Br J Urol 1993;72(1):46–51.
18. Peschers UM, Vodusek DB, Fanger G, et al. Pelvic muscle activity in nulliparous volunteers. Neurourol Urodyn 2001;20(3):269–75.
19. Yang JM, Yang SH, Huang WC. Biometry of the pubovisceral muscle and levator hiatus in nulliparous Chinese women. Ultrasound Obstet Gynecol 2006;28(5):710–6.
20. Sapsford RR, Hodges PW, Richardson CA, et al. Co-activation of the abdominal and pelvic floor muscles during voluntary exercises. Neurourol Urodyn 2001;20(1):31–42.
21. Jung SA, Pretorius DH, Padda BS, et al. Vaginal high-pressure zone assessed by dynamic 3-dimensional ultrasound images of the pelvic floor. Am J Obstet Gynecol 2007;197(1):52, e1–e7.
22. Lose L. Simultaneous recording of pressure and cross-sectional area in the female urethra: a study of urethral closure function in healthy and stress incontinent women. Neurourol Urodyn 1992;11(2):55–89.
23. Howard D, Miller JM, Delancey JO, et al. Differential effects of cough, Valsalva, and continence status on vesical neck movement. Obstet Gynecol 2000;95(4):535–40.
24. Beer-Gabel M, Teshler M, Barzilai N, et al. Dynamic transperineal ultrasound in the diagnosis of pelvic floor disorders: pilot study. Dis Colon Rectum 2002;45(2):239–45 [discussion: 245–8].
25. Weidner AC, Low VH. Imaging studies of the pelvic floor. Obstet Gynecol Clin North Am 1998;25(4):825–48, vii.
26. Healy JC, Halligan S, Reznek RH, et al. Patterns of prolapse in women with symptoms of pelvic floor weakness: assessment with MR imaging. Radiology 1997;203(1):77–81.
27. Altringer WE, Saclarides TJ, Dominguez JM, et al. Four-contrast defecography: pelvic "floor-oscopy". Dis Colon Rectum 1995;38(7):695–9.
28. Goei R, Kemerink G. Radiation dose in defecography. Radiology 1990;176(1):137–9.
29. Fielding JR, Griffiths DJ, Versi E, et al. MR imaging of pelvic floor continence mechanisms in the supine and sitting positions. AJR Am J Roentgenol 1998;171(6):1607–10.
30. Falk PM, Blatchford GJ, Cali RL, et al. Transanal ultrasound and manometry in the evaluation of fecal incontinence. Dis Colon Rectum 1994;37(5):468–72.
31. Law PJ, Bartram CI. Anal endosonography: technique and normal anatomy. Gastrointest Radiol 1989;14(4):349–53.
32. Law PJ, Kamm MA, Bartram CI. Anal endosonography in the investigation of faecal incontinence. Br J Surg 1991;78(3):312–4.
33. Law PJ, Kamm MA, Bartram CI. A comparison between electromyography and anal endosonography in mapping external anal sphincter defects. Dis Colon Rectum 1990;33(5):370–3.
34. Nichols CM, Ramakrishnan V, Gill EJ, et al. Anal incontinence in women with and those without pelvic floor disorders. Obstet Gynecol 2005;106(6):1266–71.

35. Gantke B, Schafer A, Enck P, et al. Sonographic, manometric, and myographic evaluation of the anal sphincters morphology and function. Dis Colon Rectum 1993;36(11):1037–41.
36. Gold DM, Halligan S, Kmiot WA, et al. Intraobserver and interobserver agreement in anal endosonography. Br J Surg 1999;86(3):371–5.
37. Mimura T, Kaminishi M, Kamm MA. Diagnostic evaluation of patients with faecal incontinence at a specialist institution. Dig Surg 2004;21(3):235–41 [discussion: 241].
38. Saclarides TJ. Endorectal ultrasound. Surg Clin North Am 1998;78(2):237–49.
39. Sultan AH, Kamm MA, Talbot IC, et al. Anal endosonography for identifying external sphincter defects confirmed histologically. Br J Surg 1994;81(3):463–5.
40. Deen KI, Kumar D, Williams JG, et al. Anal sphincter defects. Correlation between endoanal ultrasound and surgery. Ann Surg 1993;218(2):201–5.
41. Farouk R, Bartolo DC. The use of endoluminal ultrasound in the assessment of patients with faecal incontinence. J R Coll Surg Edinb 1994;39(5):312–8.
42. Ternent CA, Shashidharan M, Blatchford GJ, et al. Transanal ultrasound and anorectal physiology findings affecting continence after sphincteroplasty. Dis Colon Rectum 1997;40(4):462–7.
43. Savoye-Collet C, Savoye G, Koning E, et al. Anal endosonography after sphincter repair: specific patterns related to clinical outcome. Abdom Imaging 1999;24(6): 569–73.
44. Faltin DL, Boulvain M, Floris LA, et al. Diagnosis of anal sphincter tears to prevent fecal incontinence: a randomized controlled trial. Obstet Gynecol 2005;106(1): 6–13.
45. Zetterstrom JP, Mellgren A, Madoff RD, et al. Perineal body measurement improves evaluation of anterior sphincter lesions during endoanal ultrasonography. Dis Colon Rectum 1998;41(6):705–13.
46. Nielsen MB, Rasmussen OO, Pedersen JF, et al. Anal endosonographic findings in patients with obstructed defecation. Acta Radiol 1993;34(1):35–8.
47. Jackson SL, Weber AM, Hull TL, et al. Fecal incontinence in women with urinary incontinence and pelvic organ prolapse. Obstet Gynecol 1997;89(3):423–7.
48. Solomon MJ, Pager CK, Rex J, et al. Randomized, controlled trial of biofeedback with anal manometry, transanal ultrasound, or pelvic floor retraining with digital guidance alone in the treatment of mild to moderate fecal incontinence. Dis Colon Rectum 2003;46(6):703–10.
49. Kleinubing H Jr, Jannini JF, Malafaia O, et al. Transperineal ultrasonography: new method to image the anorectal region. Dis Colon Rectum 2000;43(11):1572–4.
50. Schaer GN, Koechli OR, Schuessler B, et al. Perineal ultrasound for evaluating the bladder neck in urinary stress incontinence. Obstet Gynecol 1995;85(2): 220–4.
51. Shobeiri SA, Nolan TE, Yordan-Jovet R, et al. Digital examination compared to trans-perineal ultrasound for the evaluation of anal sphincter repair. Int J Gynaecol Obstet 2002;78(1):31–6.
52. Minardi D, Parri G, d'Anzeo G. Perineal ultrasound evaluation of dysfunctional voiding in women with recurrent urinary tract infections. J Urol 2008;179(3): 947–51.
53. Poon CI, Zimmern PE. Role of three-dimensional ultrasound in assessment of women undergoing urethral bulking agent therapy. Curr Opin Obstet Gynecol 2004;16(5):411–7.
54. Timor-Tritsch IE, Platt LD. Three-dimensional ultrasound experience in obstetrics. Curr Opin Obstet Gynecol 2002;14(6):569–75.

55. Weinstein MM, Pretorius DH, Jung SA, et al. Transperineal three-dimensional ultrasound imaging for detection of anatomic defects in the anal sphincter complex muscles. Clin Gastroenterol Hepatol 2009;7(2):205–11.
56. Dietz HP, Shek C, Clarke B. Biometry of the pubovisceral muscle and levator hiatus by three-dimensional pelvic floor ultrasound. Ultrasound Obstet Gynecol 2005;25(6):580–5.
57. Sultan AH, Kamm MA, Hudson CN, et al. Anal-sphincter disruption during vaginal delivery. N Engl J Med 1993;329(26):1905–11.
58. DeLancey JO, Kearney R, Chou Q, et al. The appearance of levator ani muscle abnormalities in magnetic resonance images after vaginal delivery. Obstet Gynecol 2003;101(1):46–53.
59. Dietz HP, Lanzarone V. Levator trauma after vaginal delivery. Obstet Gynecol 2005;106(4):707–12.
60. Choi JS, Wexner SD, Nam YS, et al. Intraobserver and interobserver measurements of the anorectal angle and perineal descent in defecography. Dis Colon Rectum 2000;43(8):1121–6.
61. Padda BS, Jung SA, Pretorius D, et al. Effects of pelvic floor muscle contraction on anal canal pressure. Am J Physiol Gastrointest Liver Physiol 2007;292(2): G565–71.
62. Abdool Z, Shek KL, Dietz HP. The effect of levator avulsion on hiatal dimension and function. Am J Obstet Gynecol 2009;201(1):89, e1–e5.
63. Athanasiou S, Khullar V, Boos K, et al. Imaging the urethral sphincter with three-dimensional ultrasound. Obstet Gynecol 1999;94(2):295–301.
64. DeLancey JO. Structural aspects of the extrinsic continence mechanism. Obstet Gynecol 1988;72(3 Pt 1):296–301.
65. Bø K, Stien R. Needle EMG registration of striated urethral wall and pelvic floor muscle activity patterns during cough, Valsalva, abdominal, hip adductor, and gluteal muscle contractions in nulliparous healthy females. Neurourol Urodyn 1994;13(1):35–41.
66. Umek WH, Laml T, Stutterecker D, et al. The urethra during pelvic floor contraction: observations on three-dimensional ultrasound. Obstet Gynecol 2002;100(4): 796–800.
67. Monga AK, Robinson D, Stanton SL. Periurethral collagen injections for genuine stress incontinence: a 2-year follow-up. Br J Urol 1995;76(2):156–60.
68. Khullar V, Cardozo LD, Abbott D, et al. GAX collagen in the treatment of urinary incontinence in elderly women: a two year follow up. Br J Obstet Gynaecol 1997; 104(1):96–9.
69. Elia G, Bergman A. Periurethral collagen implant: ultrasound assessment and prediction of outcome. Int Urogynecol J Pelvic Floor Dysfunct 1996;7(6):335–8.
70. Defreitas GA, Wilson TS, Zimmern PE, et al. Three-dimensional ultrasonography: an objective outcome tool to assess collagen distribution in women with stress urinary incontinence. Urology 2003;62(2):232–6.
71. Radley SC, Chapple CR, Mitsogiannis IC, et al. Transurethral implantation of macroplastique for the treatment of female stress urinary incontinence secondary to urethral sphincter deficiency. Eur Urol 2001;39(4):383–9.
72. Dietz HP, Wilson PD. The 'iris effect': how two-dimensional and three-dimensional ultrasound can help us understand anti-incontinence procedures. Ultrasound Obstet Gynecol 2004;23(3):267–71.

Radiological Assessment of Gynecologic Malignancies

Daniel J. Bell, MBChB*, Harpreet K. Pannu, MD

KEYWORDS

- Gynecology • Computed tomography
- Magnetic resonance imaging • Ultrasonography • Sonography
- Malignancy

Patients with gynecologic malignancies are evaluated with a combination of clinical and diagnostic imaging methods. Imaging with ultrasonography (US), computed tomography (CT), and magnetic resonance (MR) has a role in detection of and characterizing gynecologic masses, and can supplement clinical staging, help in preoperative planning for surgery, and assess patients for tumor recurrence. US has a primary role in detecting and characterizing endometrial and adnexal pathology. The role of CT is primarily to stage malignancy and detect recurrence, although it can also detect larger gynecologic masses. MR imaging has added specificity over US for lesion characterization, superior contrast resolution for visualizing uterine and adnexal masses, and is also useful for staging gynecologic malignancies. This review focuses on the radiologic imaging of the 3 most common gynecologic tumors: endometrial, cervical, and ovarian carcinomas.

ENDOMETRIAL CARCINOMA

Endometrial carcinoma is the most common gynecologic malignancy, with approximately 40,000 new cases diagnosed in the United States each year.[1] Pathologically and clinically, endometrial cancer is divided into 2 main subtypes: endometrioid (Type I) and nonendometrioid (Type II) tumors. Endometrioid histology is seen in 80% to 90% of patients.[2] Patients are usually perimenopausal and have risk factors associated with increased estrogen exposure such as nulliparity, chronic anovulation, and obesity. The tumors are confined, as a rule, to the uterus and have a good

A version of this article was previously published in *PET Clinics* 5:4.

Department of Radiology, Memorial Sloan-Kettering Cancer Center, 1275 York Avenue, New York City, NY 10065, USA

* Corresponding author.

E-mail address: belld@mskcc.org

prognosis. On the other hand, nonendometrioid subtypes are seen in older multiparous women, usually without increased estrogen exposure.[3] The most common forms are uterine papillary serous carcinoma and clear cell carcinoma. These tumors have a high propensity for myometrial and vascular invasion as well as peritoneal carcinomatosis, and carry a poorer prognosis than endometrioid carcinoma.[4] Painless bleeding is the most frequent presenting symptom of endometrial cancer. Effective steps for the evaluation of patients' postmenopausal bleeding (PMB) are transvaginal sonography (TVS), endometrial biopsy (EMB), and hysteroscopy.[5] Once malignancy is detected, tumor bulk as well as local and distant spread can be assessed with imaging before surgical staging.

Role of Imaging in Primary Tumor Assessment

The role of imaging is twofold: to evaluate the symptomatic patient for a possible endometrial abnormality, and to characterize and stage disease in those with known pathology. Initial evaluation uses US to assess endometrial thickness and appearance. The normal endometrium is homogeneously hyperechoic and thin, but is thickened and heterogeneous with hyperplasia, polyps, and cancer (**Fig. 1**). The consensus statement from the Society of Radiologists in Ultrasound has defined an endometrial thickness of 5 mm or greater on TVS as being abnormal in patients with painless PMB.[5] Using a threshold of 5 mm, the sensitivity of TVS approaches that of endometrial biopsy, and had a sensitivity of 96% for detecting an endometrial abnormality in patients with cancer in a meta-analysis of 35 studies.[6] The negative predictive value (NPV) of TVS is high and can be used to obviate biopsy. However, the specificity is decreased in patients who are on hormone replacement therapy or medications such as tamoxifen. Also, endometrial thickening due to hyperplasia, polyps, fibroids, and malignancy can be difficult to distinguish on routine TVS. Presence of an echogenic lesion with a vascular stalk favors a polyp while fibroids are hypoechoic or heterogeneous and broad-based.

In equivocal cases, sonohysterography can be performed to better assess the endometrium. With this technique, the endometrial cavity is distended with saline through a small-bore catheter tip placed in the cervix while real-time TVS images of the lining are acquired to assess for smooth versus irregular thickening and masses. The endoluminal distention achieved aids in both the detection and characterization of endometrial masses. In a study of 114 patients who had an abnormal sonohysterogram, 14% had a normal-appearing endometrium on routine TVS while the sonohysterogram showed polyps and/or submucosal fibroids (**Fig. 2**).[7] Sonohysterography detected the etiology of PMB in 70% of 98 patients for an overall sensitivity of 98%, specificity of 88%, positive predictive value (PPV) of 94%, and NPV of 97%.[8] The appearance of endometrial cancer is variable, but includes thickening and a polypoid mass.[9] Using the criteria of a focal heterogeneous mass projecting into the endometrial cavity or focal thickening greater than 4 mm, a study of 88 women undergoing sonohysterography detected endometrial cancer in 8 of 9 women positive for malignancy at surgery for a sensitivity of 89%, specificity of 46%, PPV of 16%, and NPV of 97%.[10]

Once endometrial malignancy is detected, preliminary staging can be done with imaging before definitive surgical staging, which remains the standard of care for endometrial carcinoma unless the patient is a poor surgical candidate. Surgical staging involves hysterectomy, bilateral salpingo-oophorectomy, peritoneal washing, and lymphadenectomy. The key factors are the histopathologic grade of the tumor and degree of myometrial involvement. Adverse features are higher tumor grade

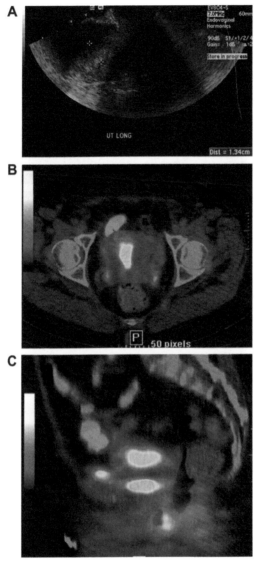

Fig. 1. Endometrioid-type endometrial carcinoma in a 70-year-old woman with breast carcinoma following an incidental finding of an ^{18}F-fluorodeoxyglucose (FDG)-avid endometrium on PET/CT performed at staging. (*A*) Longitudinal transvaginal sonogram of the uterus shows the diffusely thickened endometrium. PET/CT (*B*) axial and (*C*) sagittal images show an FDG-avid focus in the endometrium.

and deep myometrial invasion, as these are associated with higher stage disease such as nodal metastases.

Of the imaging modalities available, MR imaging has excellent contrast resolution and allows assessment of the entire pelvis in multiple planes without the use of ionizing radiation. The role of MR imaging is primarily to stage endometrial cancer. In unusual cases it can be also a supplemental technique to evaluate the endometrium if US or

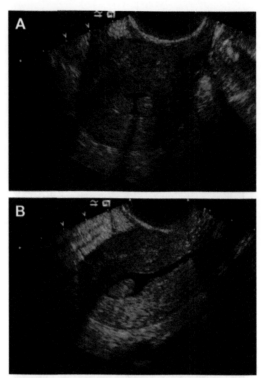

Fig. 2. Endometrial polyps in a 40-year-old woman with breast carcinoma. (*A*) Transverse and (*B*) longitudinal sonohysterogram demonstrates the presence of 2 echogenic endometrial polyps.

hysteroscopy cannot be performed or are equivocal. The T2-weighted and contrast-enhanced sequences are the most useful for distinguishing normal endometrium and myometrium from disease. Imaging parallel and perpendicular to the plane of the uterus optimizes visualization of the endometrial-myometrial interface. The normal endometrium is hyperintense on T2-weighted images while tumors tend to be interme-diate and heterogeneous in signal intensity (**Fig. 3**).[11] Hemorrhage in the endometrial cavity can also have low signal intensity on T2 but is hyperintense on precontrast T1-weighted images. Compared with tumors, the inner myometrium or junctional zone is hypointense on T2-weighted images. The junctional zone is more conspicuous in premenopausal women but is not well seen in older postmenopausal women. Because of this limiting factor, contrast-enhanced scans have been found to be more useful because after injection of contrast the tumor enhances less than the normal myometrium and is relatively hypointense.[12,13] Invasive disease appears as a hypointense tumor extending into the myometrium, with irregularity and disruption of the enhancing inner myometrium at the endometrial-myometrial interface.

The staging system for endometrial carcinoma was revised by the International Federation of Gynecology and Obstetrics (FIGO) in 2008 (**Table 1**). Tumors confined to the endometrium or having less than 50% depth of myometrial invasion are defined as Stage IA while those with 50% or more myometrial invasion are Stage IB.[14] MR imaging can assess the degree of myometrial involvement and distinguish superficial from deep invasion with a relatively high accuracy of 83% to 89%.[15–17] In a study of

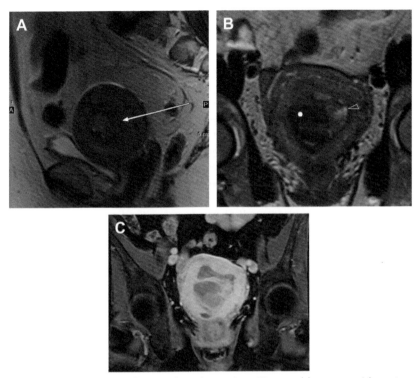

Fig. 3. Endometrioid-type endometrial carcinoma in a 60-year-old woman with postmenopausal bleeding. (*A*) Sagittal T2-weighted, (*B*) coronal T2-weighted, and (*C*) coronal T1-weighted fat-saturation post-gadolinium MR imaging show an enhancing polypoid endometrial mass in the left side of the fundus (*arrow* in *A*, *arrowhead* in *B*) without deep myometrial invasion. Adjacent fibroid (*white circle*) is also noted.

101 patients, including 48 with pathologic evidence of deep myometrial invasion, 90% of patients were correctly staged by MR imaging and 10% were understaged.[18] Assessment of invasion can be difficult in the presence of coexisting benign myometrial abnormalities such as adenomyosis, as well as in patients with an indistinct junctional zone, if there is poor contrast between the tumor and normal myometrium or if tumor involves the uterine cornua.[12,19] Adenomyosis appears as heterogeneous ill-defined regions with thickening of the junctional zone and small cystic foci on T2-weighted images. The addition of dynamic contrast-enhanced images to T2-weighted images increased the accuracy for depth of myometrial invasion from 78% to 92% in a study on 50 patients.[19,20] The likelihood ratios (LR) for predicting deep myometrial invasion with contrast-enhanced MR imaging were positive LR of 10.11 and negative LR of 0.1 in a meta-analysis of 9 articles with a total of 742 patients.[21]

In addition to the myometrium, cervical stromal invasion is also evaluated on MR imaging, as it is an indication for radical hysterectomy.[4] The normal cervical stroma is hypointense on T2-weighted images and is replaced by intermediate signal intensity tumor in cases of invasion. Endocervical extension manifests as widening of the cervical canal by an inferiorly extending endometrial mass. Addition of intravenous contrast can improve detection of cervical invasion. One study has reported that

Table 1	
FIGO staging of endometrial carcinoma	
I	Tumor confined to corpus uteri
IA	Tumor limited to endometrium or invades less than one-half of the myometrium
IB	Tumor invades one-half or more of the myometrium
II	Tumor invades cervical stroma but does not extend beyond uterus[a]
III	Local and/or regional tumor spread
IIIA	Tumor invades serosa of corpus uteri and/or adnexae
IIIB	Vaginal and/or parametrial involvement
IIIC	Metastases to pelvic and/or para-aortic nodes
IIIC1	Positive pelvic nodes
IIIC2	Positive para-aortic nodes
IV	Tumor invades bladder and/or bowel mucosa and/or distant metastases
IVA	Tumor invades bladder and/or bowel mucosa
IVB	Distant metastases

[a] Endocervical glandular involvement without stromal invasion is considered as Stage I.

From Pecorelli S. Revised FIGO staging for carcinoma of the vulva, cervix, and endometrium. Int J Gynaecol Obstet 2009;105:103–4.

MR imaging had 80% sensitivity, 96% specificity, 89% PPV, and 93% NPV for assessing cervical infiltration.[15] The new FIGO classification places endocervical glandular tumor extension into Stage I and cervical stromal invasion into Stage II.[14] With local extension of tumor beyond the uterus, there is abnormal intermediate T2 signal intensity tissue in the parametrial fat or adnexae. Loss of the normal low signal intensity wall on T2-weighted images suggests bladder or rectal invasion.[4]

Recently, there has been interest in applying diffusion-weighted imaging (DWI) to evaluate gynecologic malignancies including endometrial cancer. DWI is a noncontrast technique that assesses the random motion of water molecules in tissue. The resultant information can be qualitatively assessed or quantified by calculating the apparent diffusion coefficient (ADC) value. The "b" value or factor determines the strength of the diffusion weighting on the image. In tissues with mobile molecules such as vessels, the ADC value is high and the diffusion or motion of water results in a visual decrease in signal intensity. Conversely, in tissues with high cellularity such as tumors, the movement of water is restricted resulting in a low ADC value and high visual signal intensity. Endometrial cancer shows restricted diffusion appearing hyperintense on high b value ($b = 1000$ s/mm^2) images.[22,23] Combining DWI with T2-weighted images may aid in the detection of tumors.[24] The ADC values of tumor are reported to be lower than benign endometrial pathology or the normal endometrium.[22,23,25] A trend for higher grade tumors to demonstrate lower ADC values compared with those of lower grade ones has been described as well.[23,25] DWI can help supplement the contrast-enhanced scan for myometrial invasion. In a study of 62 patients with endometrial cancer, Rechichi and colleagues[26] reported a sensitivity of 84.6% and specificity of 70.6% for DWI for depicting myometrial invasion. However, a lower accuracy of DWI compared with contrast-enhanced MR imaging has also been reported because of lower spatial resolution of DWI.[22,25] Other limitations of DWI include image degradation due to magnetic field inhomogeneity and motion artifacts and poor background signal on high b-value images. Fusion of DWI with T2-weighted images aids in anatomic localization. Normal endometrium can also have restricted diffusion, and the cutoff ADC values for distinguishing normal from cancerous tissue are not established at present.[23]

MR imaging has superior soft tissue contrast and therefore is the main imaging modality for staging endometrial cancer, with TVS and CT as alternatives if MR imaging is not available. A meta-analysis of 6 CT, 16 US, and 25 MR imaging studies showed superiority of contrast-enhanced MR imaging for myometrial invasion.[27] Endometrial/myometrial echogenicity and vascularity as well as regularity of the endometrial-myometrial interface are assessed on US.[28] Newer techniques such as contrast-enhanced and 3-dimensional US may prove helpful for endometrial cancer.[29] In a study of 35 patients with endometrial cancer, tumor conspicuity increased following injection of contrast, and a feeding vessel was seen in 77% of patients.[30] Time-intensity curves of tumor enhancement can be also generated. CT provides a rapid assessment and global overview of the abdomen and pelvis for distant metastases, and is usually readily available. Soft tissue contrast resolution of CT is lower than that of MR imaging but spatial resolution tends to be higher. Evaluation of myometrial invasion was initially hampered by imaging limited to the axial plane, while the lie of the uterus was variable and usually not perpendicular to the axial plane.[31] Current multidetector-row CT (MDCT) scanners have made thin slices, isotropic datasets, and reconstruction in multiple user-defined planes possible. Using multiplanar reconstructions and imaging 70 seconds after contrast injection on a 16-row MDCT scanner, the depth of myometrial invasion was correctly assessed in 18 of 21 patients with endometrial cancer.[32]

Role of Imaging for Assessment of Nodal and Distant Metastases, and Recurrence

Nodal metastases from endometrial cancer involve pelvic and para-aortic nodes. Tumors from the middle and inferior uterus drain to the parametrial and obturator nodes whereas those from the proximal body and fundus drain to the common iliac and para-aortic nodes.[12] Lymphatic drainage from the uterus also occurs to obturator nodes, and tumor can spread via the round ligament to inguinal nodes as well. The likelihood of nodal spread increases in the presence of greater than 50% invasion of the myometrium compared with those with lesser amount of invasion.[19] In addition to depth of myometrial invasion, the incidence of nodal disease is also linked to the tumor histologic grade. For patients with greater than 50% myometrial extension, nodal metastases occurred in 28% of those with grade 3 tumors in a series of 349 patients undergoing pelvic lymphadenectomy.[33] Lymphadenectomy is associated with morbidity, and therefore a combination of preoperative imaging and intraoperative evaluation is helpful in determining if this surgical procedure is indeed necessary in each patient.[19,34] Imaging findings suggestive of nodal involvement include a short-axis diameter greater than 1 cm and presence of necrosis.[4] However, size criteria have a wide range of sensitivities, and the addition of other techniques such as lymph node contrast agents or DWI may be helpful.[35,36] Recurrent disease occurs at the vagina, abdominal and pelvic nodes, peritoneum, and lung. MR imaging can evaluate for local disease while CT is used for surveillance.

CERVICAL CARCINOMA

Cervical carcinoma is the third most common gynecologic cancer, with an estimated 11,000 cases of invasive cancer in the United States in 2009. Incidence and mortality rates have declined over the past several decades because of screening and detection of preinvasive cervical lesions.[1] Approximately 85% of cases are squamous cell carcinoma and most of the remainder are adenocarcinoma. Uncommon subtypes include adenosquamous carcinoma, lymphoma, adenoma malignum, and small cell carcinoma, the latter tending to be locally invasive as well to have distant metastases.

Role of Imaging in Primary Tumor Assessment

Unlike endometrial cancer, the recommended staging of cervical carcinoma is clinical by physical examination, colposcopy, examination under anesthesia, non–cross-sectional imaging studies such as chest radiography, barium enema, and intravenous urography, and by endoscopic studies such as cystoscopy and rectosigmoidoscopy (**Table 2**). Patients are triaged to surgical or nonsurgical management based on initial staging results. Clinical staging can under- or overstage patients because nodal status is not determined and parametrial assessment is limited.[37] Physical examination is also subject to interobserver variability, and discrepancies between clinical staging and surgery range from 25% in early-stage to 65% in advanced-stage disease.[38] Therefore, there has been interest in assessing the additional value of cross-sectional imaging for parametrial invasion, metastatic pelvic nodes, distant metastases, and overall improved staging of cervical cancer. If MR imaging, CT, and PET/ CT are available, they can be incorporated into patient staging.

Lesion size, extension into the uterine corpus, depth of stromal invasion, parametrial spread, and pelvic adenopathy are evaluated on imaging. The primary tumor, uterine anatomy, and cervical anatomy are better seen on MR imaging due to high soft tissue contrast, whereas nodes and distant metastases are seen on both CT and MR

Table 2
FIGO staging of cervical carcinoma

I	Cervical carcinoma confined to cervix (extension to corpus disregarded)
IA	Invasive carcinoma diagnosed only by microscopy
IA1	Measured stromal invasion 3.0 mm or less in depth and 7.0 mm or less in horizontal spread
IA2	Measured stromal invasion more than 3.0 mm but less than 5.0 mm in depth with a horizontal spread 7.0 mm or less
IB	Clinically visible lesion confined to the cervix or preclinical lesion greater than Stage IA[a]
IB1	Clinically visible lesion 4.0 cm or less in greatest dimension
IB2	Clinically visible lesion more than 4.0 cm in greatest dimension
II	Cervical carcinoma invades beyond uterus but not to pelvic wall or to lower third of vagina
IIA	Tumor without parametrial invasion
IIA1	Clinically visible lesion 4.0 cm or less in greatest dimension
IIA2	Clinically visible lesion more than 4.0 cm in greatest dimension
IIB	Tumor with obvious parametrial invasion
III	Tumor extends to pelvic wall and/or involves lower third of vagina, and/or causes hydronephrosis or nonfunctioning kidney
IIIA	Tumor involves lower third of vagina, no extension to pelvic wall
IIIB	Tumor extends to pelvic wall and/or causes hydronephrosis or nonfunctioning kidney
IV	Cancer extends beyond true pelvis or biopsy proof of invasion of the bladder or rectal mucosa
IVA	Tumor spread to adjacent organs
IVB	Distant metastases

[a] All macroscopically visible lesions, even with superficial invasion, are Stage IB.
From Pecorelli S. Revised FIGO staging for carcinoma of the vulva, cervix, and endometrium. Int J Gynaecol Obstet 2009;105:103–4.

imaging. Including images perpendicular to the endocervical canal provides a cross section of the cervix and aids in diagnosing parametrial extension. The critical distinction is between stages I and IIA, which are treated surgically, and advanced disease, stage IIB and higher, which is treated with radiation or combined chemoradiation.

On MR imaging, the primary tumor is intermediate in signal intensity on T2-weighted images and is hyperintense relative to the hypointense normal cervical stroma. Tumors can be exophytic, infiltrating, or endocervical with a barrel shape. Endovaginal and multiphase imaging following intravenous contrast may aid in the visualization of small tumors.[39,40] The margins of the tumor relative to the lower uterine segment myometrium, internal and external cervical os, and vaginal fornices are determined. Next, the integrity of the cervical stroma is assessed. An intact ring of hypointense tissue on T2-weighted images has a high NPV for parametrial invasion (**Fig. 4**). Disruption of the stromal ring, contour irregularity, and vessel abutment are suspicious for parametrial disease (**Fig. 5**) which, however, can be difficult to assess in the presence of bulky masses and full-thickness invasion of the cervical stroma. Gross parametrial mass and ureteral encasement are definitive for tumor extension (**Fig. 6**).

On CT small primary tumors are typically isodense to the cervix whereas large ones can be hypodense, heterogeneous, and necrotic. Gross parametrial spread and

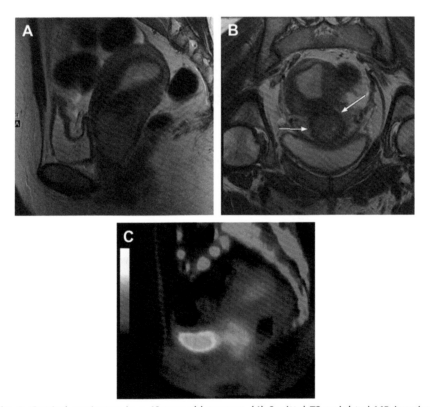

Fig. 4. Cervical carcinoma in a 40-year-old woman. (*A*) Sagittal T2-weighted MR imaging shows a bulky tumor extending from the external to internal os. (*B*) Coronal T2-weighted image demonstrates thinning of the low signal intensity cervical stroma (*arrows*) but no gross disruption to suggest parametrial invasion. (*C*) Sagittal PET/CT image shows FDG avidity of the cervical lesion.

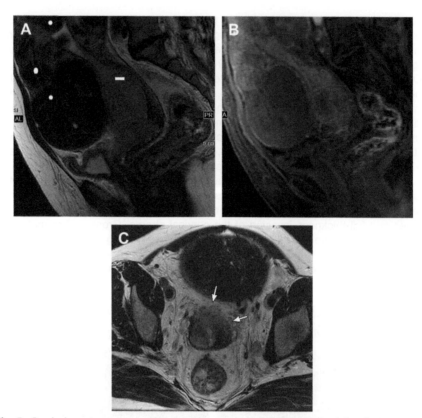

Fig. 5. Cervical carcinoma in a 50-year-old woman. (*A*) Sagittal T2-weighted MR imaging shows a bulky cervical mass (*white rectangle*) of intermediate T2 signal intensity compared with the fibroids of low signal intensity (*white circles*). The tumor extends into the upper vagina. (*B*) Sagittal T1-weighted fat-saturation post-gadolinium image shows enhancement of the cervical mass. (*C*) On the axial T2-weighted image the normal T2 low signal intensity fibrous stroma is absent (*arrows*) and there is contour irregularity suspicious for parametrial invasion.

ureteral obstruction are similar as for MR imaging. Tumors within 3 mm of the pelvic side wall, encasement of the iliac vessels, and muscle enlargement indicate pelvic side-wall invasion. Preservation of the normal fat plane between the bladder and rectum excludes involvement while tumor abutment or abnormal wall signal intensity are suspicious for disease.

Numerous studies have evaluated the utility of MR imaging and CT for staging the local extent of cervical cancer, with variable results. A retrospective review of the medical records of 255 patients imaged between 1992 and 2003 found clinical pelvic examination to be superior to MR imaging and CT, and had a higher sensitivity and specificity for parametrial disease.[41] However, over recent years these imaging modalities have evolved technologically and other investigators have reported relatively high accuracy for staging with MR imaging.[37,42,43] A recent study evaluating the depth of stromal invasion with MR imaging in 53 patients with stage I or IIA disease found an agreement of 75% between MR imaging and pathology for tumor infiltration of greater or less than 50% of the width of the cervical stroma.[44] The NPV of MR

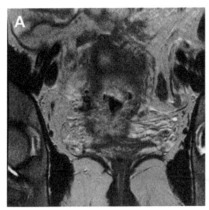
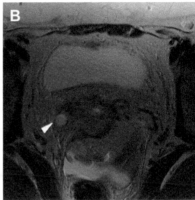

Fig. 6. Cervical carcinoma in a 45-year-old woman. (*A*) Coronal and (*B*) axial T2-weighted MR imaging shows a bulky heterogeneous cervical mass with invasion of the cervical stroma. There is dilatation of the adjacent distal right ureter (*arrowhead*) secondary to parametrial invasion.

imaging for parametrial invasion is high. In a study on 113 patients comparing MR imaging and surgery, the NPV was 95% and the PPV 67%.[42] Microscopic disease can cause false-negative results while parametrial inflammation and stranding can lead to a false-positive diagnosis. A high sensitivity of 80% and specificity of 91% for parametrial invasion has been found with MR imaging using an endovaginal imaging coil.[40] Sensitivities and specificities of 67% to 87% and 79% to 92% have been reported for involvement of the vaginal fornices when compared with surgery.[42,44] A meta-analysis of 57 MR imaging and/or CT articles published between 1985 and 2002 found a higher sensitivity for MR imaging than with CT for parametrial invasion (74% vs 55%), with equivalent specificities.[38] MR imaging also had a higher sensitivity and specificity for bladder invasion. The utility of CT and MR imaging has been assessed in a series of articles by the American College of Radiology Imaging Network (ACRIN) and Gynecologic Oncology Group (GOG).[45–48] A multicenter study by both groups compared MR imaging, CT, and clinical staging in patients with early-stage cervical cancer imaged between 2000 and 2002, and found a lower sensitivity and specificity for disease extent compared with results from single-institution studies. MR imaging had the highest agreement with pathology for tumor size and involvement of the uterine corpus.[46] Detection of parametrial invasion and reader agreement was also higher for MR imaging than for CT.[48] For detecting malignancies of stage IIB or higher, both MR imaging and CT had a low sensitivity (42% for CT, 53% for MR imaging) but high specificity (82% for CT, 74% for MR imaging) and NPV (84% for CT, 85% for MR imaging).[45]

Areas where imaging can potentially impact on patient management are the evaluation of young patients for possible trachelectomy, assessment of tumor volume, and tumor response to therapy. Trachelectomy involves resection of the cervix and upper 1- to 2-cm of vagina and parametrium, with preservation of the uterine corpus for future fertility in patients of reproductive age with stage I cervical cancer.[49] The uterine corpus is incised from the cervix approximately 5 mm below the internal os, the resected cervix is assessed for a tumor-free margin, and the uterine body is sutured to the upper vagina. Location of the cervical tumor margin relative to the internal os and lower uterine segment myometrium is helpful in determining if the patient is

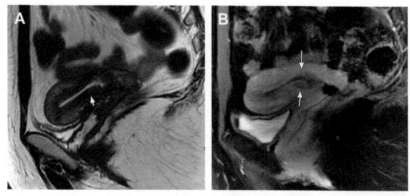

Fig. 7. Cervical carcinoma in a 35-year-old woman who was initially considered for trache-lectomy. (*A*) Sagittal T2-weighted and (*B*) sagittal T1-weighted fat-saturation post-gadolinium MR imaging shows endocervical tumor up to the internal os. There is abnormal signal intensity (*arrows*) in the anterior cervical stroma with extension to the junctional zone of the anterior lower uterine segment. Trachelectomy was attempted but the cervical margin was positive for tumor, and the patient underwent hysterectomy.

a candidate for this procedure (**Fig. 7**). A waist in the uterine contour, differences in the signal intensity of the cervical stroma relative to the myometrium, and location of the uterine vessels have been used to define the location of the internal os on imaging.[50] A study by 2 experienced readers found that the internal os was visible on MR imaging in most patients, with good interobserver variability for estimating the distance of the tumor from the internal os.[51] High sensitivity and specificity of MR imaging for tumor involvement of the internal os as compared with surgery has also been reported.[44] Retrospective analysis of MR imaging in 150 patients found a sensitivity of 90%, specificity of 98%, PPV of 86%, and NPV of 98% for tumor extension to internal os.[43]

In addition to staging, the appearance of the cervical tumor on imaging may be helpful in predicting patient response to nonsurgical therapy and outcome. Tumor volume before and after treatment can be calculated from the largest-diameter measurements on multiplanar images and may help as a prognostic indicator in these patients.[52]

Dynamic contrast-enhanced MR imaging is also an exciting new method to assess tumor angiogenesis and perfusion of cervical cancer before and after therapy. The contrast agent diffuses into the extravascular space, with no linear relationship between the concentration of gadolinium and the resultant tissue signal. The degree of enhancement is related to a combination of blood flow, vascular permeability, and volume of extracellular space. Semiquantitative parameters obtained by plotting tissue signal intensity over time depend on machine and imaging parameters. Quantitative analysis using pharmacokinetic modeling provides parameters such as the transfer constant between blood plasma and the extravascular extracellular space, and the volume of the extravascular extracellular space.[53] Increased tumor enhancement suggests increased vascularity and oxygenation, which may indicate increased radiosensitivity and delivery of therapeutic drugs. Dynamic contrast-enhanced MR imaging has been performed in patients with cervical cancer before and during radiation and has been shown to predict response to therapy and disease-free survival.[54–58]

DWI also has the potential to demonstrate the primary tumor in cervical cancer and response to treatment.[59,60] Cervical cancer has a lower ADC value than that of the normal epithelium. ADC values have been noted to increase with treatment.[59–61]

Role of Imaging for Assessment of Nodal and Distant Metastases, and Recurrence

Nodal disease is not assessed in the clinical FIGO staging system but does influence patient prognosis. Tumor can initially spread to the external iliac, internal iliac, and pre-sacral nodes, followed by the common iliac and para-aortic nodes.[62] The extent of lymphadenectomy and radiation field may need to be increased if para-aortic nodes are suspicious for metastatic involvement. As for other tumors, findings suggestive of nodal tumor include a short-axis diameter greater than 1 cm and the presence of necrosis. Size criteria are, however, not reliable.[63] In the ACRIN/GOG trial, sensitivity was low for both MR imaging and CT (37% and 31%) but specificity was high (94% and 86%).[45] The prediction of nodal involvement on MR imaging was higher than for CT when combined with results for tumor size.[47] A 10-year review of 150 patients with early-stage cervical cancer at a single institution also found similar sensitivity and specificity for nodal metastases with MR imaging.[43] Sensitivity slightly improves but specificity decreases when the short-axis diameter cutoff for distinguishing normal from abnormal nodes is decreased from 1 cm to 0.5 cm.[44] A meta-analysis of 57 MR imaging and/or CT articles reported a sensitivity of 60% for MR imaging and 43% for CT with equivalent specificity.[38] Another meta-analysis that included PET found that on a per-patient basis, PET or PET/CT had higher sensitivity (82%) compared with CT (50%) or MR imaging (56%), with all 3 having specificities of greater than 90%. On a region or node based basis, sensitivity was in a similar range with 54% for PET, 52% for CT, and 38% for MR imaging.[64] The addition of DWI or lymph node contrast agents to MR imaging has been suggested.[65] Ultrasmall superparamagnetic iron oxide (USPIO) particles are taken up by macrophages in nodes resulting in a loss of signal on gradient echo sequences. However, in metastatic nodes there is replacement of the normal nodal architecture by tumor, resulting in diminished macrophages and lack of significant signal loss. This method can increase the sensitivity of MR imaging for identifying nodal metastases.[66]

Recurrent cervical cancer occurs mainly in the pelvis in the vaginal vault, parametrium, and pelvic side wall. Distant metastases occur in the peritoneum, liver, adrenal glands, lungs, and bones.[66] Local recurrence is better evaluated with MR imaging, whereas CT is used in search of distant sites. Posttreatment changes can be difficult to distinguish from residual or recurrent tumor, as inflammation can show increased signal on T2-weighted images and enhancement similar to tumor.

OVARIAN CARCINOMA

Ovarian carcinoma is the second most frequent gynecologic malignancy in the United States with approximately 20,000 new cases annually. About two-thirds of patients present with advanced FIGO Stage III or IV disease. Ovarian cancer accounts for a greater number of deaths than all other gynecologic malignancies.[1,67] The World Health Organization subdivides ovarian tumors into 3 main types based on the cell of origin: epithelial, sex-cord stromal, and germ cell tumors.[68] Epithelial tumors account for approximately 90% of ovarian cancers and can have serous, mucinous, endometrioid, clear cell, and undifferentiated histologies.[69,70] Serous carcinoma represents approximately 80% of all ovarian cancers and is histologically graded as low or high grade. Low-grade serous carcinomas arise from borderline tumors whereas high-grade tumors do not have a definite precursor lesion, are more frequent, and have a poorer prognosis. Borderline tumors lack stromal invasion and occur at a younger age group than invasive cancer. Primary ovarian mucinous carcinoma is uncommon and is diagnosed after excluding metastatic disease to the ovary.

Role of Imaging in Primary Tumor Assessment

Imaging is used to characterize an adnexal mass and assess for metastatic disease following the diagnosis of malignancy. US is the first-line approach for lesion characterization, with MR imaging a problem-solving tool. CT or MR imaging can be used to stage patients for metastatic disease. Adnexal lesions are common findings on imaging procedures, and the key is to distinguish benign from potentially malignant lesions.

Functional cysts occur in premenopausal women, and cysts are also seen in approximately 20% of postmenopausal women. Short-term follow-up imaging is helpful to distinguish functional from pathologic cystic lesions. Benign lesions include corpus luteum cysts, endometriomas, dermoids, and hydrosalpinx. Feature analysis is used to determine the likelihood of a benign lesion that need only be followed, or of indeterminate or malignant lesions that require resection.[67,71] Simple cysts are anechoic on US with increased through transmission and no internal soft tissue. Sonographic, CT, and MR imaging criteria suspicious for malignancy include the presence of a vascular soft tissue component. This component can further consist of septations greater than 3 mm in thickness, papillary projections, or nodules (**Figs. 8–10**).[72] A retracted blood clot, fibrin strands, and dermoid plug are benign causes of soft tissue nodularity. Assessment of nodule echogenicity and color Doppler imaging for internal vascularity are helpful.[72,73] Combining Doppler with gray-scale imaging improves the

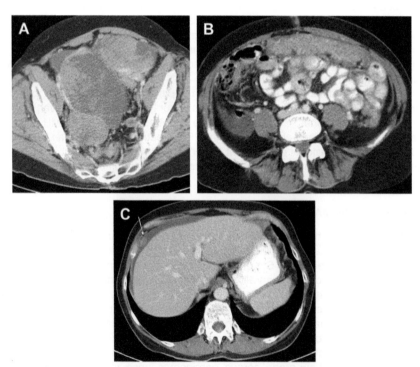

Fig. 8. High-grade serous ovarian carcinoma in a 70-year-old woman with a pelvic mass and elevated serum CA125 level. Intravenous and oral contrast-enhanced axial CT images demonstrate (*A*) bilateral heterogeneous enhancing adnexal masses in the pelvis, (*B*) anterior omental cake and small amount of ascites in the mid-abdomen, and (*C*) a peritoneal deposit (*arrow*) adjacent to the liver.

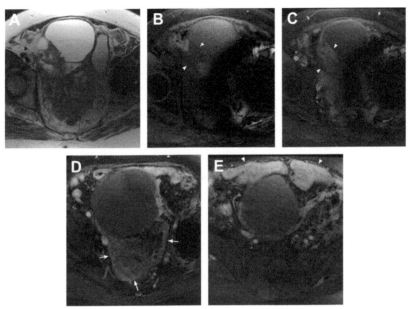

Fig. 9. Ovarian carcinoma in an 80-year-old woman with prior hysterectomy. (*A*) Axial T2-weighted, (*B*) axial T1-weighted fat-saturation precontrast, and (*C*) axial T1-weighted fat-saturation post-gadolinium MR imaging show a complex cystic ovarian mass with an enhancing solid component (*arrowheads*). (*D* and *E*) Axial T1-weighted fat-saturation post-gadolinium images at more superior levels demonstrate enhancing serosal disease involving the bowel (*arrows* in *D*) and omental tissue (*arrowheads* in *E*). Susceptibility artifact from left hip replacement is noted in the left pelvis.

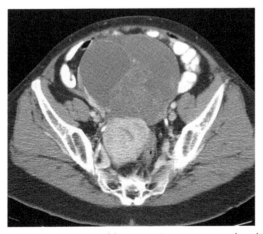

Fig. 10. Ovarian metastasis in a 50-year-old woman. Intravenous and oral contrast-enhanced axial CT through the pelvis shows a multiseptate midline cystic mass, histologically proven as metastasis from a mucinous adenocarcinoma of the pancreatic tail (not shown).

diagnostic assessment of ovarian lesions. A meta-analysis of 46 studies compared the relative utility of gray-scale imaging, color Doppler, and Doppler flow analysis for interrogating adnexal masses, and found that the combination of these methods was more powerful than their individual use.[74] Although US and MR imaging are both highly sensitive for adnexal lesions, MR imaging is more specific for characterization of fat and blood products. MR imaging can also evaluate solid components in large lesions that may be difficult to entirely visualize on US. In a study of 103 women with sonographic features worrisome for adnexal malignancy, MR imaging and US both had a sensitivity of greater than 80% for malignancy but the specificity for MR imaging, 84%, was much higher than for US, 59%, due to the ability of MR imaging to accurately define benign lesions such as dermoid, endometrioma, and fibroid.[67,75] Increased specificity can affect patient management and may obviate the need for surgery.[76] A meta-analysis showed that in a patient with a sonographically indeterminate adnexal lesion, the posttest probability of malignancy increased with the addition of MR imaging and, to a lesser extent, CT.[77] In a review of 143 patients with CT and histopathology, features suspicious for malignancy in cystic lesions included multilocularity, irregular wall thickening, and soft tissue nodules, while unilocular homogeneous lesions with thin walls and smooth contour tended to be benign.[71] Secondary findings of implants, ascites, and other metastases also aid in distinguishing malignant from benign lesions.

In addition to the traditional feature analysis method of evaluating adnexal lesions, there have been reports on applying contrast-enhanced US and dynamic contrast-enhanced MR imaging for these masses. In sonographic studies of patients who were imaged for 3 to 5 minutes after contrast injection, malignancies have had a slower washout of contrast than benign lesions.[78–80] The development of diagnostic criteria for the kinetics of contrast enhancement may increase the specificity of US for adnexal malignancies.[80] Malignancies have a faster time to peak and greater enhancement on dynamic contrast-enhanced MR imaging than benign lesions.[81] A report correlating dynamic MR imaging with histology found a positive correlation between the slope of the enhancement curve and tumor expression of vascular endothelial growth factor receptor, which plays a role in angiogenesis.[81] DWI also provides tissue perfusion information at low b values, and the vascular signal intensity has been preliminarily investigated in the primary tumor and abdominal metastases of advanced epithelial ovarian cancer.[82]

Ovarian carcinoma is staged surgically with exploratory laparotomy, oophorectomy, hysterectomy, omentectomy, and peritoneal washings, as well as inspection and resection of abdominal and pelvic implants (**Table 3**). The goal of surgery is to optimally debulk patients to deposits of residual disease less than 1 cm in size. Tumor spreads to the contralateral ovary, uterus, and peritoneum. Cells are carried up into the abdomen by the peritoneal fluid that normally circulates from the pelvis to the abdomen along a clockwise pathway—initially to the right paracolic gutter, the right upper quadrant around the liver and diaphragm, and thence to the greater omentum and left paracolic gutter. Implants are therefore usually found in the cul-de-sac, paracolic and subphrenic spaces, greater omentum, and on the surfaces of the liver, bowel, and spleen.[68,70,73,83,84] Preoperative CT or MR imaging can be used to determine the extent of disease.[68] Metastatic implants appear as discrete nodules, masses, nodularity, or plaque-like thickening on the surface of viscera, and can enhance.[85,86] Implants on the liver and spleen can cause scalloping of the surface. Protrusion of the implant into the liver with irregularity of the interface suggests invasion of the parenchyma by tumor, which may require more extensive resection.[87]

Table 3	
FIGO staging of ovarian carcinoma	
I	Tumor limited to ovary
IA	Tumor limited to one ovary with intact capsule and no tumor on ovarian surface. No tumor cells in ascites or peritoneal washings
IB	Tumor limited to both ovaries with intact capsule and no tumor on ovarian surface. No tumor cells in ascites or peritoneal washings
IC	Tumor limited to one or both ovaries with: ruptured capsule or tumor on ovarian surface or tumor cells in ascites or peritoneal washings
II	Ovarian tumor with pelvic extension and/or implants
IIA	Extension and/or implants on fallopian tube(s) and/or uterus No tumor cells in ascites or peritoneal washings
IIB	Extension to and/or implants on other pelvic soft tissues No tumor cells in ascites or peritoneal washings
IIC	Extension to and/or implants on pelvic soft tissues with tumor cells in ascites or peritoneal washings
III	Peritoneal metastases outside the pelvis
IIIA	Microscopic peritoneal metastasis beyond pelvis
IIIB	Macroscopic (≤ 2 cm) peritoneal metastasis beyond pelvis
IIIC	Macroscopic (>2 cm) peritoneal metastasis beyond pelvis and/or metastasis to regional nodes
IV	Distant metastasis

Note: Liver capsule metastases are Stage III and liver parenchymal metastases are Stage IV.
From Mironov S, Akin O, Pandit-Taskar N, et al. Ovarian cancer. Radiol Clin North Am 2007;45:56.

MR imaging and CT perform similarly in the preoperative staging of ovarian carcinoma.[75,84,88,89] Staging is primarily done with CT because of its shorter imaging time and ready availability. Sensitivity is higher for lesions larger than 1 to 2 cm as well as for those surrounded by ascitic fluid. CT is more sensitive than MR imaging for calcified implants. In a study on 64 patients scanned with CT slice thickness of 5 to 10 mm, sensitivity was lower for subcentimeter implants, 25% to 50%, as compared with overall sensitivity of 85% to 93% for peritoneal disease.[90] Thinner slices are possible with current MDCT scanners, and multiplanar images have an incremental value over axial images for detecting metastases.[91] Sensitivity and specificity on CT and MR imaging can also depend on the lesion location, paracolic gutters versus diaphragm.[86,91] Small implants on the bowel are particularly difficult to detect with CT and MR imaging but can have greater conspicuity on PET/CT. A recent study on 133 patients with ovarian masses found a sensitivity of 94% and specificity of 71% for CT or MR imaging for diagnosis of extraovarian abdominopelvic metastases, whereas PET/CT had a higher specificity of 83% for a similar sensitivity.[92] The addition of the DWI sequence to MR imaging improved the sensitivity for peritoneal metastases in 34 patients with ovarian and non-ovarian cancers from 73% to 90% while specificity remained similar, at 90%.[93]

Pelvic sites of disease are easily assessed and debulked at surgery. However, resection of tumors in the upper abdomen can be more difficult, and preoperative imaging can help in the surgical planning for locations such as the lesser sac, porta hepatis, diaphragm, and mesentery. Parenchymal liver metastases also need to be distinguished from surface implants (**Figs. 11** and **12**). In a study of 137 women with a new diagnosis of ovarian carcinoma, CT and MR imaging were equally able to

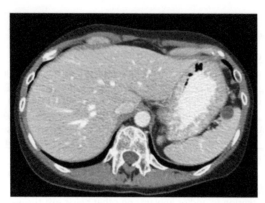

Fig. 11. Serous ovarian carcinoma in a 60-year-old woman. Intravenous and oral contrast-enhanced axial CT through the upper abdomen shows a cystic splenic surface metastatic implant.

predict which patients were less likely to have effective cytoreduction, with sensitivity, specificity, PPV, and NPV of 76%, 99%, 94%, and 96%, respectively.[94]

Role of Imaging for Assessment of Nodal and Distant Metastases and Recurrence

The peritoneal route of dissemination is the most common for ovarian cancer, with lymphatic and hematogenous metastases being less common. Pelvic nodal metastases occur following tumor spread via the broad ligament. Para-aortic nodes can be involved by tumor spread along the gonadal vessels.[70] Supradiaphragmatic lymph node metastases can be also found.[68] Size criteria are used to assess nodes similar to other malignancies. Hematogenous metastases are least common and as a rule involve the liver, lung, and pleura.[70,73] Treated patients are followed by serial CA125 assays and CT or MR imaging of the abdomen and pelvis. PET/CT can be helpful in the presence of rising tumor markers with no obvious disease on CT. Recurrence occurs typically in the peritoneal cavity, lymph nodes, abdominal viscera, and thorax,[95,96] and can be identified for preoperative planning. In a series of 36 patients

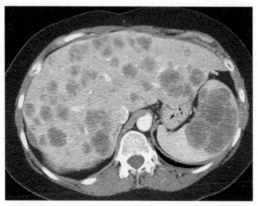

Fig. 12. Ovarian carcinoma in a 50-year-old woman. Intravenous and oral contrast-enhanced axial CT through the upper abdomen demonstrates multiple parenchymal liver and splenic metastases.

with recurrent ovarian cancer, the presence of pelvic side-wall invasion at CT was predictive of suboptimal secondary cytoreduction.[88]

SUMMARY

Initial assessment of patients with symptoms suspicious for gynecologic malignancy is performed with US, using MR imaging as a problem-solving tool for indeterminate lesions. Local staging of uterine malignancies is primarily done with MR imaging whereas ovarian malignancies are typically staged by CT. Morphologic imaging features are used primarily for distinguishing benign from malignant gynecologic masses and for evaluating potential metastatic disease. Newer tools such as DWI and dynamic contrast-enhanced imaging may result in improved lesion characterization and staging.

REFERENCES

1. American Cancer Society. Cancer facts and figures. Atlanta (GA): American Cancer Society; 2009.
2. Mendivil A, Schuler KM, Gehrig PA. Non-endometrioid adenocarcinoma of the uterine corpus: a review of selected histological subtypes. Cancer Control 2009;16:46–52.
3. Prat J, Gallardo A, Cuatrecasas M, et al. Endometrial carcinoma: pathology and genetics. Pathology 2007;39:72–87.
4. Peungjesada S, Bhosale PR, Balachandran A, et al. Magnetic resonance imaging of endometrial carcinoma. J Comput Assist Tomogr 2009;33:601–8.
5. Goldstein RB, Bree RL, Benson CB, et al. Evaluation of the woman with postmenopausal bleeding: Society of Radiologists in Ultrasound-Sponsored Consensus Conference statement. J Ultrasound Med 2001;20:1025–36.
6. Smith-Bindman R, Kerlikowske K, Feldstein VA, et al. Endovaginal ultrasound to exclude endometrial cancer and other endometrial abnormalities. JAMA 1998; 280:1510–7.
7. Laifer-Narin S, Ragavendra N, Parmenter EK, et al. False-normal appearance of the endometrium on conventional transvaginal sonography: comparison with saline hysterosonography. AJR Am J Roentgenol 2002;178:129–33.
8. Bree RL, Bowerman RA, Bohm-Velez M, et al. US evaluation of the uterus in patients with postmenopausal bleeding: a positive effect on diagnostic decision making. Radiology 2000;216:260–4.
9. Davidson KG, Dubinsky TJ. Ultrasonographic evaluation of the endometrium in postmenopausal vaginal bleeding. Radiol Clin North Am 2003;41:769–80.
10. Dubinsky TJ, Stroehlein K, Abu-Ghazzeh Y, et al. Prediction of benign and malignant endometrial disease: hysterosonographic-pathologic correlation. Radiology 1999;210:393–7.
11. Frei KA, Kinkel K. Staging endometrial cancer: role of magnetic resonance imaging. J Magn Reson Imaging 2001;13:850–5.
12. Manfredi R, Gui B, Maresca G, et al. Endometrial cancer: magnetic resonance imaging. Abdom Imaging 2005;30:626–36.
13. Saez F, Urresola A, Larena JA, et al. Endometrial carcinoma: assessment of myometrial invasion with plain and gadolinium-enhanced MR imaging. J Magn Reson Imaging 2000;12:460–6.
14. Creasman W. Revised FIGO staging for carcinoma of the endometrium. Int J Gynaecol Obstet 2009;105:109.

15. Manfredi R, Mirk P, Maresca G, et al. Local-regional staging of endometrial carcinoma: role of MR imaging in surgical planning. Radiology 2004;231:372–8.
16. Chung HH, Kang SB, Cho JY, et al. Accuracy of MR imaging for the prediction of myometrial invasion of endometrial carcinoma. Gynecol Oncol 2007;104:654–9.
17. Nakao Y, Yokoyama M, Hara K, et al. MR imaging in endometrial carcinoma as a diagnostic tool for the absence of myometrial invasion. Gynecol Oncol 2006; 102:343–7.
18. Félix A, Cunha TM. Preoperative assessment of deep myometrial and cervical invasion in endometrial carcinoma: comparison of magnetic resonance imaging and histopathologic evaluation. J Obstet Gynaecol 2007;27:65–70.
19. Sala E, Crawford R, Senior E, et al. Added value of dynamic contrast-enhanced magnetic resonance imaging in predicting advanced stage disease in patients with endometrial carcinoma. Int J Gynecol Cancer 2009;19:141–6.
20. Utsunomiya D, Notsute S, Hayashida Y, et al. Endometrial carcinoma in adenomyosis: assessment of myometrial invasion on T2-weighted spin-echo and gadolinium-enhanced T1-weighted images. AJR Am J Roentgenol 2004;182: 399–404.
21. Frei KA, Kinkel K, Bonᵉl HM, et al. Prediction of deep myometrial invasion in patients with endometrial cancer: clinical utility of contrast-enhanced MR imaging-a meta-analysis and Bayesian analysis. Radiology 2000;216:444–9.
22. Shen SH, Chiou YY, Wang JH, et al. Diffusion-weighted single-shot echo-planar imaging with parallel technique in assessment of endometrial cancer. AJR Am J Roentgenol 2008;190:481–8.
23. Tamai K, Koyama T, Saga T, et al. Diffusion-weighted MR imaging of uterine endometrial cancer. J Magn Reson Imaging 2007;26:682–7.
24. Inada Y, Matsuki M, Nakai G, et al. Body diffusion-weighted MR imaging of uterine endometrial cancer: is it helpful in the detection of cancer in nonenhanced MR imaging? Eur J Radiol 2009;70:122–7.
25. Takeuchi M, Matsuzaki K, Nishitani H. Diffusion-weighted magnetic resonance imaging of endometrial cancer: differentiation from benign endometrial lesions and preoperative assessment of myometrial invasion. Acta Radiol 2009;50: 947–53.
26. Rechichi G, Galimberti S, Signorelli M, et al. Myometrial invasion in endometrial cancer: diagnostic performance of diffusion-weighted MR imaging at 1.5-T. Eur Radiol 2010;20:754–62.
27. Kinkel K, Kaji Y, Yu KK, et al. Radiologic staging in patients with endometrial cancer: a meta-analysis. Radiology 1999;212:711–8.
28. Ozdemir S, Celik C, Emlik D, et al. Assessment of myometrial invasion in endometrial cancer by transvaginal sonography, Doppler ultrasonography, magnetic resonance imaging and frozen section. Int J Gynecol Cancer 2009;19:1085–90.
29. Alcázar JL, Galván R, Albela S, et al. Assessing myometrial infiltration by endometrial cancer: uterine virtual navigation with three-dimensional US. Radiology 2009;250:776–83.
30. Song Y, Yang J, Liu Z, et al. Preoperative evaluation of endometrial carcinoma by contrast-enhanced ultrasonography. BJOG 2009;116:294–8 [discussion: 298–9].
31. Hardesty LA, Sumkin JH, Hakim C, et al. The ability of helical CT to preoperatively stage endometrial carcinoma. AJR Am J Roentgenol 2001;176:603–6.
32. Tsili AC, Tsampoulas C, Dalkalitsis N, et al. Local staging of endometrial carcinoma: role of multidetector CT. Eur Radiol 2008;18:1043–8.
33. Chi DS, Barakat RR, Palayekar MJ, et al. The incidence of pelvic lymph node metastasis by FIGO staging for patients with adequately surgically staged

endometrial adenocarcinoma of endometrioid histology. Int J Gynecol Cancer 2008;18:269–73.

34. Celik C, Ozdemir S, Esen H, et al. The clinical value of preoperative and intraoperative assessments in the management of endometrial cancer. Int J Gynecol Cancer 2010;20:358–62.

35. Namimoto T, Awai K, Nakaura T, et al. Role of diffusion-weighted imaging in the diagnosis of gynecological diseases. Eur Radiol 2009;19:745–60.

36. Lin G, Ng KK, Chang CJ, et al. Myometrial invasion in endometrial cancer: diagnostic accuracy of diffusion-weighted 3.0-T MR imaging—initial experience. Radiology 2009;250:784–92.

37. Ozsarlak O, Tjalma W, Schepens E, et al. The correlation of preoperative CT, MR imaging, and clinical staging (FIGO) with histopathology findings in primary cervical carcinoma. Eur Radiol 2003;13:2338–45.

38. Bipat S, Glas AS, van der Velden J, et al. Computed tomography and magnetic resonance imaging in staging of uterine cervical carcinoma: a systematic review. Gynecol Oncol 2003;91:59–66.

39. Seki H, Azumi R, Kimura M, et al. Stromal invasion by carcinoma of the cervix: assessment by dynamic MR imaging. AJR Am J Roentgenol 1997;168:1579–85.

40. deSouza NM, Dina R, McIndoe GA, et al. Cervical cancer: value of an endovaginal coil magnetic resonance imaging technique in detecting small volume disease and assessing parametrial extension. Gynecol Oncol 2006;102:80–5.

41. Hancke K, Heilmann V, Straka P, et al. Pretreatment staging of cervical cancer: is imaging better than palpation?: role of CT and MRI in preoperative staging of cervical cancer: single institution results for 255 patients. Ann Surg Oncol 2008;15:2856–61.

42. Choi SH, Kim SH, Choi HJ, et al. Preoperative magnetic resonance imaging staging of uterine cervical carcinoma: results of prospective study. J Comput Assist Tomogr 2004;28:620–7.

43. Sahdev A, Sohaib SA, Wenaden AE, et al. The performance of magnetic resonance imaging in early cervical carcinoma: a long-term experience. Int J Gynecol Cancer 2007;17:629–36.

44. Manfredi R, Gui B, Giovanzana A, et al. Localized cervical cancer (stage <IIB): accuracy of MR imaging in planning less extensive surgery. Radiol Med 2009; 114:960–75.

45. Hricak H, Gatsonis C, Chi DS, et al. Role of imaging in pretreatment evaluation of early invasive cervical cancer: results of the intergroup study American College of Radiology Imaging Network 6651-Gynecologic Oncology Group 183. J Clin Oncol 2005;23:9329–37.

46. Mitchell DG, Snyder B, Coakley F, et al. Early invasive cervical cancer: tumor delineation by magnetic resonance imaging, computed tomography, and clinical examination, verified by pathologic results, in the ACRIN 6651/GOG 183 Intergroup Study. J Clin Oncol 2006;24:5687–94.

47. Mitchell DG, Snyder B, Coakley F, et al. Early invasive cervical cancer: MRI and CT predictors of lymphatic metastases in the ACRIN 6651/GOG 183 intergroup study. Gynecol Oncol 2009;112:95–103.

48. Hricak H, Gatsonis C, Coakley FV, et al. Early invasive cervical cancer: CT and MR imaging in preoperative evaluation—ACRIN/GOG comparative study of diagnostic performance and interobserver variability. Radiology 2007;245:491–8.

49. Abu-Rustum NR, Sonoda Y, Black D, et al. Fertility-sparing radical abdominal trachelectomy for cervical carcinoma: technique and review of the literature. Gynecol Oncol 2006;103:807–13.

50. Peppercorn PD, Jeyarajah AR, Woolas R, et al. Role of MR imaging in the selection of patients with early cervical carcinoma for fertility-preserving surgery: initial experience. Radiology 1999;212:395–9.
51. Bipat S, van den Berg RA, van der Velden J, et al. The role of magnetic resonance imaging in determining the proximal extension of early stage cervical cancer to the internal os. Eur J Radiol 2009. [Epub ahead of print].
52. Lee DW, Kim YT, Kim JH, et al. Clinical significance of tumor volume and lymph node involvement assessed by MRI in stage IIB cervical cancer patients treated with concurrent chemoradiation therapy. J Gynecol Oncol 2010;21:18–23.
53. Tofts PS, Brix G, Buckley DL, et al. Estimating kinetic parameters from dynamic contrast-enhanced T(1)-weighted MRI of a diffusible tracer: standardized quantities and symbols. J Magn Reson Imaging 1999;10:223–32.
54. Yuh WT, Mayr NA, Jarjoura D, et al. Predicting control of primary tumor and survival by DCE MRI during early therapy in cervical cancer. Invest Radiol 2009;44:343–50.
55. Mayr NA, Wang JZ, Zhang D, et al. Longitudinal changes in tumor perfusion pattern during the radiation therapy course and its clinical impact in cervical cancer. Int J Radiat Oncol Biol Phys 2010;77:502–8.
56. Zahra MA, Tan LT, Priest AN, et al. Semiquantitative and quantitative dynamic contrast-enhanced magnetic resonance imaging measurements predict radiation response in cervix cancer. Int J Radiat Oncol Biol Phys 2009;74:766–73.
57. Semple SI, Harry VN, Parkin DE, et al. A combined pharmacokinetic and radiologic assessment of dynamic contrast-enhanced magnetic resonance imaging predicts response to chemoradiation in locally advanced cervical cancer. Int J Radiat Oncol Biol Phys 2009;75:611–7.
58. Donaldson SB, Buckley DL, O'Connor JP. Enhancing fraction measured using dynamic contrast-enhanced MRI predicts disease-free survival in patients with carcinoma of the cervix. Br J Cancer 2010;102:23–6.
59. Messiou C, Morgan VA, De Silva SS, et al. Diffusion weighted imaging of the uterus: regional ADC variation with oral contraceptive usage and comparison with cervical cancer. Acta Radiol 2009;50:696–701.
60. Liu Y, Bai R, Sun H, et al. Diffusion-weighted imaging in predicting and monitoring the response of uterine cervical cancer to combined chemoradiation. Clin Radiol 2009;64:1067–74.
61. Payne GS, Schmidt M, Morgan VA, et al. Evaluation of magnetic resonance diffusion and spectroscopy measurements as predictive biomarkers in stage 1 cervical cancer. Gynecol Oncol 2010;116(2):246–52.
62. Park JM, Charnsangavej C, Yoshimitsu K, et al. Pathways of nodal metastasis from pelvic tumors: CT demonstration. Radiographics 1994;14(6):1309–21.
63. Yang WT, Man Lam WW, Yu MY, et al. Comparison of dynamic helical CT and dynamic MR imaging in the evaluation of pelvic lymph nodes in cervical carcinoma. AJR Am J Roentgenol 2000;175:759–66.
64. Choi HJ, Ju W, Myung SK, et al. Diagnostic performance of computer tomography, magnetic resonance imaging, and positron emission tomography or positron emission tomography/computer tomography for detection of metastatic lymph nodes in patients with cervical cancer: meta-analysis. Cancer Sci 2010; 101:1471–9.
65. Lin G, Ho KC, Wang JJ, et al. Detection of lymph node metastasis in cervical and uterine cancers by diffusion-weighted magnetic resonance imaging at 3T. J Magn Reson Imaging 2008;28:128–35.

66. Sala E, Wakely S, Senior E, et al. MRI of malignant neoplasms of the uterine corpus and cervix. AJR Am J Roentgenol 2007;188:1577–87.
67. Rieber A, Nussle K, Stohr I, et al. Preoperative diagnosis of ovarian tumors with MR imaging: comparison with transvaginal sonography, positron emission tomography, and histologic findings AJR. Am J Roentgenol 2001;177:123–9.
68. Edge SB, Byrd DR, Compton CC, et al, editors. AJCC cancer staging handbook. 7th edition. New York: Springer; 2010.
69. Iyer VR, Lee SI. MRI, CT and PET/CT for ovarian cancer detection and adnexal lesion characterization. AJR Am J Roentgenol 2010;194:311–21.
70. Mironov S, Akin O, Pandit-Taskar N, et al. Ovarian cancer. Radiol Clin North Am 2007;45:149–66.
71. Zhang J, Mironov S, Hricak H, et al. Characterization of adnexal masses using feature analysis at contrast-enhanced helical computed tomography. J Comput Assist Tomogr 2008;32:533–40.
72. Brown DL, Dudiak KM, Laing FC. Adnexal masses: US characterization and reporting. Radiology 2010;254:342–54.
73. Shaaban A, Rezvani M. Ovarian cancer: detection and radiologic staging. Clin Obstet Gynecol 2009;52:73–93.
74. Kinkel K, Hricak H, Lu Ying, et al. US characterization of ovarian masses: a meta-analysis. Radiology 2000;217:803–11.
75. Kurtz AB, Tsimikas JV, Tempany CM, et al. Diagnosis and staging of ovarian cancer: comparative values of Doppler and conventional US, CT, and MR imaging correlated with surgery and histopathologic analysis—report of the Radiology Diagnostic Oncology Group. Radiology 1999;212:19–27.
76. Spencer JA, Forstner R, Cunha TM, et al. ESUR Female Imaging Sub-Committee. ESUR guidelines for MR imaging of the sonographically indeterminate adnexal mass: an algorithmic approach. Eur Radiol 2010;20:25–35.
77. Kinkel K, Lu Y, Mehdizade A, et al. Indeterminate ovarian mass at US: incremental value of second imaging test for characterization—meta-analysis and Bayesian analysis. Radiology 2005;236:85–94.
78. Ordén MR, Jurvelin JS, Kirkinen PP. Kinetics of a US contrast agent in benign and malignant adnexal tumors. Radiology 2003;226:405–10.
79. Marret H, Sauget S, Giraudeau B, et al. Contrast-enhanced sonography helps in discrimination of benign from malignant adnexal masses. J Ultrasound Med 2004;23:1629–39.
80. Fleischer AC, Lyshchik A, Jones HW 3rd, et al. Diagnostic parameters to differentiate benign from malignant ovarian masses with contrast-enhanced transvaginal sonography. J Ultrasound Med 2009;28:1273–780.
81. Thomassin-Naggara I, Bazot M, Daraï E, et al. Epithelial ovarian tumors: value of dynamic contrast-enhanced MR imaging and correlation with tumor angiogenesis. Radiology 2008;248:148–59.
82. Sala E, Priest AN, Kataoka M, et al. Apparent diffusion coefficient and vascular signal fraction measurements with magnetic resonance imaging: feasibility in metastatic ovarian cancer at 3 Tesla: technical development. Eur Radiol 2010;20:491–6.
83. Coakley FV, Hricak H. Imaging of peritoneal and mesenteric disease: key concepts for the clinical radiologist. Clin Radiol 1999;54:563–74.
84. Tempany CMC, Zou KH, Silverman SG, et al. Staging of advanced ovarian cancer: comparison of imaging modalities—report from the Radiological Diagnostic Oncology Group. Radiology 2000;215:761–7.

85. Forstner R, Hricak H, Occhipinti KA, et al. Ovarian cancer: staging with CT and MR imaging. Radiology 1995;197:619–26.

86. Ricke J, Sehouli J, Hach C, et al. Prospective evaluation of contrast-enhanced MRI in the depiction of peritoneal spread in primary or recurrent ovarian cancer. Eur Radiol 2003;13:943–9.

87. Akin O, Sala E, Moskowitz CS, et al. Perihepatic metastases from ovarian cancer: sensitivity and specificity of CT for the detection of metastases with and those without liver parenchymal invasion. Radiology 2008;248:511–7.

88. Funt SA, Hricak H, Abu-Rustum N, et al. Role of CT in the management of recurrent ovarian cancer. AJR Am J Roentgenol 2004;182:393–8.

89. Pecorelli S. Revised FIGO staging for carcinoma of the vulva, cervix, and endometrium. Int J Gynaecol Obstet 2009;105:103–4.

90. Coakley FV, Choi PH, Gougoutas CA, et al. Peritoneal metastases: detection with spiral CT in patients with ovarian cancer. Radiology 2002;223:495–9.

91. Pannu HK, Horton KM, Fishman EK. Thin section dual-phase multidetector-row computed tomography detection of peritoneal metastases in gynecologic cancers. J Comput Assist Tomogr 2003;27:333–40.

92. Nam EJ, Yun MJ, Oh YT, et al. Diagnosis and staging of primary ovarian cancer: correlation between PET/CT, Doppler US, and CT or MRI. Gynecol Oncol 2010; 116:389–94.

93. Low RN, Sebrechts CP, Barone RM, et al. Diffusion-weighted MRI of peritoneal tumors: comparison with conventional MRI and surgical and histopathologic findings—a feasibility study. AJR Am J Roentgenol 2009;193:461–70.

94. Qayyum A, Coakley FV, Westphalen AC, et al. Role of CT and MR imaging in predicting optimal cytoreduction of newly diagnosed primary epithelial ovarian cancer. Gynecol Oncol 2005;96:301–6.

95. Park CM, Kim SH, Kim SH, et al. Recurrent ovarian malignancy: patterns and spectrum of imaging findings. Abdom Imaging 2003;28:404–15.

96. Sahdev A, Hughes JH, Barwick T, et al. Computed tomography features of recurrent ovarian carcinoma according to time to relapse. Acta Radiol 2007;48: 1038–44.

Ultrasound for Pelvic Pain II: Nongynecologic Causes

Susan J. Ackerman, MD*, Abid Irshad, MD, Munazza Anis, MD

KEYWORDS

• Appendicitis • Diverticulitis • Mesenteric adenitis
• Ureteral calculus • Bowel obstruction
• Inflammatory bowel disease

Acute pelvic pain in women is a common presenting complaint that can result from various conditions. Because these conditions can be of gynecologic or nongynecologic origin, they may pose a challenge to the diagnostic acumen of physicians, including radiologists. A thorough workup should include clinical history, physical examination, laboratory data, and appropriate imaging studies, all of which should be available to the radiologist for evaluation. Ultrasound is the primary imaging modality in women with acute pelvic pain because of its high sensitivity, low cost, wide availability, and lack of ionizing radiation, particularly when a gynecologic disorder is suspected as the underlying cause. However, other modalities such as computed tomography (CT) and magnetic resonance imaging (MRI) may be very helpful, especially when a nongynecologic condition is suspected.

Nongynecologic causes of acute pelvic pain include appendicitis, diverticulitis, ureteral calculi, mesenteric adenitis, bowel obstruction, inflammatory bowel disease, and metastatic disease.

APPENDICITIS

Appendicitis is one of the most common nongynecologic causes of acute pelvic pain and right lower quadrant pain. Typically, these patients also present with nausea, vomiting, and anorexia. Physical examination and laboratory test results usually show abdominal tenderness and leukocytosis. However, the diagnosis can often be made on clinical evaluation alone. Ultrasound, CT, and MRI have proven to be useful examinations in avoiding unnecessary surgeries, especially in patients with atypical clinical presentations, particularly when the appendix is located at an unusual position,

A version of this article was previously published in *Ultrasound Clinics* 5:2.
Department of Radiology and Radiological Sciences, Medical University of South Carolina, 96 Jonathan Lucas Street, Charleston, SC 29425, USA
* Corresponding author.
E-mail address: ackerman@musc.edu

Obstet Gynecol Clin N Am 38 (2011) 69–83
doi:10.1016/j.ogc.2011.02.004
0889-8545/11/$ – see front matter © 2011 Elsevier Inc. All rights reserved.

such as retrocecal, retroileal, or pericolic gutter (15% of cases)[1] or located behind a gravid uterus. Negative laparotomy findings have been reported in 35% to 45% of women of reproductive age who were suspected to have appendicitis.[2] When the clinical picture is unclear, the imaging can not only aid in the diagnosis but also reduce the frequency of unnecessary surgical intervention.

Ultrasound compares favorably with CT in diagnosing appendicitis, with sensitivities of 75% to 90% and specificities of 86% to 100%. A positive diagnosis can be made when a distended, noncompressible tubular blind-ending structure with a wall-to-wall diameter greater than 7 mm is visible or if the individual wall is greater than 3 mm in thickness (**Figs. 1** and **2**).[3,4] In the transverse section, the inflamed appendix usually appears as a double concentric ring like a target sign. Although an inflamed appendix is noncompressible, the inflamed bowel can also be noncompressible. One can use graded compression to displace normal gas-containing loops of bowel to get a better look at the structure. Identifying the appendix in its entirety is important because appendicitis can be limited to the distal end.

Other findings suggesting appendicitis include inflammation of the adjacent mesenteric or omental fat and a shadowing appendicolith (see **Fig. 2**). In appendices measuring 5 to 7 mm, the diagnosis may be confirmed by the nonuniformity of the mural wall layers and the presence of increased blood flow in the appendix on color Doppler imaging. Once an inflamed appendix has been identified, ultrasound has a high specificity for diagnosing acute appendicitis.

However, the spontaneous resolution of appendicitis among other factors may contribute negatively toward its specificity.[5] Ultrasound may just show localized free fluid in the periappendiceal region when the appendix is not clearly seen on ultrasound, such as in cases of advanced-stage pregnancy (**Fig. 3**A, B). In these cases, a noncontrast MR (T2-weighted sequence) may be used for further evaluation (**Fig. 3**C, D). A periappendiceal abscess will appear on ultrasound as a hypoechoic fluid collection and may display a mass effect. Inflamed bowel may be difficult to distinguish from acute appendicitis, but can be differentiated through assessing the

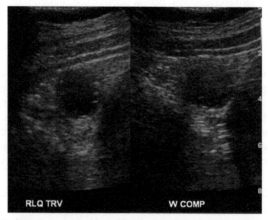

RLQ TRV   W COMP

Fig. 1. Appendicitis showing non compressibility. Two transverse ultrasouns images through the right lower quadrant obtained without compression (*left image*) and with transducer compression (*right image*) show the appendix as a rounded fluid-filled structure. This structure is noncompressible because it shows no significant change in shape or height between images without and with compression. (*From* Angle R, Irshad A, Ackerman S. Practical imaging of acute pelvic pain in premenopausal women. Contemp Diagn Radiol 2010; 33(1):4; with permission.)

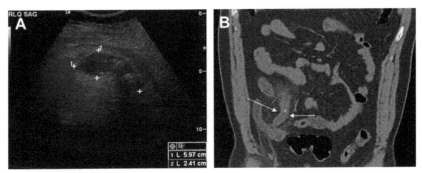

Fig. 2. Appendicitis with appendicolith. (*A*) Utrasound image through the right lower quadrant showing a fluid-filled elongated structure (*calipers*). This structure is 2.4 cm thick and contains internal fluid, debris, and calcifications, suggesting appendicolith. (*B*) Noncontrast coronal CT slice through the abdomen of the same patient showing a dilated appendix (*arrows*) with internal calcification. Moderate fat stranding is noted around the appendix, suggesting periappendiceal inflammation. (*From* Angle R, Irshad A, Ackerman S. Practical imaging of acute pelvic pain in premenopausal women. Contemp Diagn Radiol 2010; 33(1):4; with permission.)

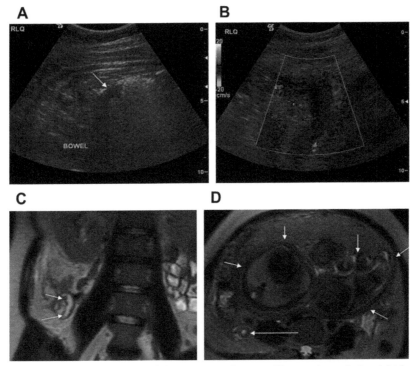

Fig. 3. Appendicitis in pregnancy. (*A*) Transverse ultrasound image through the right lower quadrant showing an anechoic triangular fluid pocket between the bowel loops (*arrow*). (*B*) Color Doppler image through the same area showing fluid adjacent to the vessels. (*C*) T2-weighted coronal MR image through the abdomen showing fluid-filled thickened appendix (*arrows*) with mild stranding in the fat. (*D*) Axial T2-weighted image showing a fluid-filled thickened appendix (*long arrow*). A fetus is noted in the central abdomen (*small arrows*).

maximum thickening of the muscle layer of adjacent bowel and the appearance of the mucosal/submucosal complex.[6]

When the appendix is not visualized at all, the radiologist should carefully review the cecal tip and iliac vessels before reporting the study as normal. Limitation of sonography in diagnosing acute appendicitis could be secondary to an unusual location of the appendix (such as a retrocecal location), ruptured appendicitis, and obesity.[7] Additionally, a gas-filled appendix may be mistaken for small bowel, or a perforated appendix may become deflated. Occasionally, the inflammation may resolve secondary to spontaneous movement of the appendicolith relieving the obstruction.

DIVERTICULITIS

Diverticulitis is the inflammation of an outpouching of the colon. Left-sided diverticulosis is marked by multiplicity, associated muscular hypertrophy, and dysfunction, whereas right-sided diverticuli are predominantly solitary. It usually presents with symptoms of fever, anorexia, lower abdominal/pelvic pain, and obstination. Like epiploic appendagitis, it usually occurs in the left lower quadrant but can occur in the right lower quadrant.

The role of imaging is primarily to distinguish diverticulitis from other entities and to assess its severity to determine if surgery or interventional management will be required. Although CT is the preferred imaging modality for diverticulitis, ultrasound can also aid in the diagnosis. Endovaginal sonography can be particularly useful in diagnosing diverticulitis if it involves the pelvis. Endorectal or endovaginal scanning for diagnosing diverticulitis has shown the sensitivity of sonography to be approximately 94%.[8,9]

Three sonographic findings are generally used to diagnose diverticulitis: a segmental area of thickened bowel wall, an inflamed diverticulum, and inflamed pericolic fat. Abscesses and fistulas can also be seen with ultrasound. Although bowel wall thickening can be asymmetric, it usually retains its normal three layers. Preservation of the colonic wall layers distinguishes uncomplicated diverticulitis from cancer of the colon.[7] An inflamed diverticulum is visible as either a hypoechoic or hyperechoic outpouching of the bowel wall surrounded by a hypoechoic border. The diverticulum may contain gas or a fecalith, and therefore dirty or clean shadowing may be associated (**Fig. 4**). The pericolic fat will appear as a hyperchoic tissue adjacent to the bowel

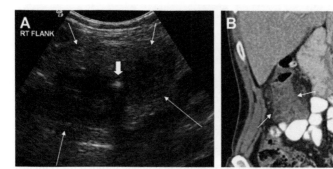

Fig. 4. Diverticulitis. (*A*) Transverse ultrasound image through the right flank that shows a thick-walled structure (*arrows*) in the area of the ascending colon. A small amount of fluid is present in the lumen with calcification suggestive of fecalith (*thick arrow*). (*B*) Coronal slice of a contrast-enhanced CT scan through the abdomen showing a thickened ascending colon (*arrows*). A few diverticuli with fat stranding are seen in the surrounding tissue.

wall around the inflamed diverticulum. Although abscesses generally appear as hypo-echoic masses, they may also be hyperechoic. The fistulas generally appear as hypo-echoic bands.[10]

URETERAL CALCULUS

Women with ureteral calculi typically present with flank pain that radiates to the ipsi-lateral groin and vulva. Commonly, the patient will have hematuria, dysuria, and urgency. CT is currently the preferred imaging modality in the evaluation of renal colic. Ultrasound may not be sensitive for detecting ureteral calculi but is still considered very useful in evaluating ureteral obstruction because of its high sensitivity to detect hydronephrosis (**Fig. 5**). Yilmaz and colleagues[11] showed that although ultrasound had a specificity of 97%, it only had a sensitivity of 19% for detecting ureteral calculi. However, they did not include transvaginal sonography in their study. In comparison, the same study showed the sensitivity and specificity of a noncontrast spiral CT to be 97% and 94%, respectively.

In another study by Patlas and colleagues, ultrasound showed a 93% sensitivity and 95% specificity for diagnosing ureteral calculi.[12] Distal ureteric stones close to the ure-terovesical junction may be seen easily on ultrasound secondary to improved visibility of the distal ureteric regions when using the bladder as a window (**Fig. 6**A, C). A ureteral calculus is seen as an echogenic focus that shows posterior acoustic shadowing. Ultra-sound has a special role in evaluating acute pain in pregnant women.[6] Transvaginal ultrasound can also be useful in detecting ureterovesical junction stones; however,

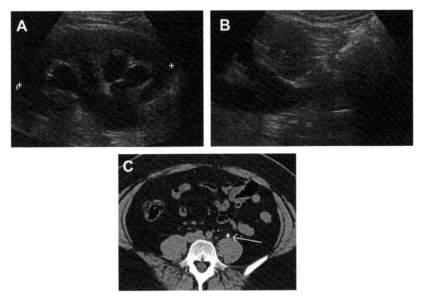

Fig. 5. Left mid ureteric calculus. (*A*) Ultrasound image through the left kidney showing moderate hydronephrosis. (*B*) Sagittal image through the left proximal ureter showing dilated upper ureter. The mid ureter is obscured by the bowel gas. (*C*) Axial slice of a non-contrast CT scan through the lower abdomen of the same patient that shows a small calculus (*arrow*) in the line of left mid ureter. (*From* Angle R, Irshad A, Ackerman S. Practical imaging of acute pelvic pain in premenopausal women. Contemp Diagn Radiol 2010;33(1):4; with permission.)

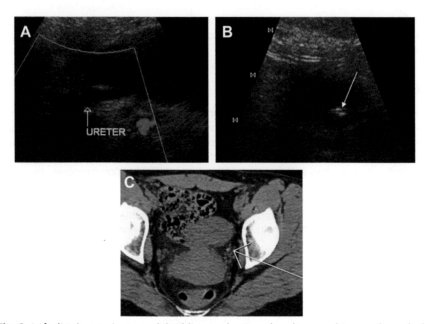

Fig. 6. Left distal ureteric stone. (*A*) Oblique color Doppler ultrasound image through the distal left ureter and bladder showing dilated left distal ureter (*arrow*). (*B*) Transverse image through the urinary bladder showing a small echogenic focus (*arrow*) in the area of the left distal ureter/ureterovesical junction with posterior acoustic shadowing suggestive of a stone. (*C*) Noncontrast CT scan; axial slice through the pelvis shows a small calcific density in the area of the left distal ureter (*arrow*) consistent with distal ureteric stone. (*From* Angle R, Irshad A, Ackerman S. Practical imaging of acute pelvic pain in premenopausal women. Contemp Diagn Radiol 2010;33(1); with permission.)

the remainder of the ureter is usually difficult to assess secondary to bowel gas. In the early phase of acute ureteral obstruction, the hydronephrosis may not be evident and the calculus may not be visible. However, one may see indirect signs of acute ureteral obstruction, including perirenal fluid, abnormally increased echotexture of the central renal sinus, and elevation of the arterial resistive index in the affected kidney. Asymmetry in the ureteral jets, with absent or less-frequent ureteral jet on the affected side, has also been identified with ureteral obstruction.[13]

Although appendicitis, diverticulitis, and ureteral calculus are some of the more common nongynecologic causes of pelvic pain, other less-common entities should also be considered. These entities include mesenteric adenitis, epiploic appendagitis, enteric duplications cysts, inguinal hernia, hydrocele, and bowel obstruction.

MESENTERIC ADENITIS

High-frequency transducers in the evaluation of lower abdominal pain may be able to detect enlarged abdominal lymph nodes. The term *mesenteric lymphadenitis* is used to describe an inflammatory process of the abdominal lymph nodes when the sole finding is enlarged lymph nodes and the patient presents with abdominal pain. It is usually a self-limiting process. A recent study by Simanovsky and Hiller[14] reports that enlarged abdominal lymph nodes of 10 mm or greater in the short axis in the clinical setting of abdominal pain may represent mesenteric lymphadenitis (**Fig. 7**).

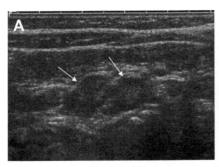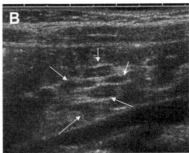

Fig. 7. Mesenteric adenitis. (A) Transverse ultrasound image through the right lower abdomen showing two adjacent lobulated masses (arrows). These masses show internal echogenic areas consistent with lymph nodes. (B) Transverse ultrasound image through the lower abdomen also shows multiple prominent lymph nodes (arrows) within the mesenteric fat as shown by surrounding echogenic areas. (Courtesy of Dr Jeanne Hill.)

Although mesenteric adenitis is predominantly seen in the pediatric population, it can occur in adults as a cause of lower quadrant/pelvic pain. In the pediatric literature, *mesenteric adenitis* is a term used for specific inflammation of mesenteric lymph nodes, caused by *Yersinia*, *Staphylococcus*, *Salmonella*, and other types of mycobacteria and viruses.[14] In the older population, multiple enlarged pelvic or mesenteric lymph nodes may occur in malignancy, appendicitis, or other inflammatory bowel conditions.

EPIPLOIC APPENDAGITIS

Epiploic appendagitis usually occurs on the left side but can mimic appendicitis when it occurs in the right lower quadrant. Epiploic appendages are visceral peritoneal outpouchings containing fat and blood vessels. Normally these appendages are invisible at sonography because their density is similar to that of surrounding fatty tissue. Epiploic appendagitis occurs from ischemia, inflammation, or spontaneous torsion of an epiploic appendage of the large bowel. The most common clinical presentation is pelvic pain in young patients after strenuous exercise or stretching. Typically, the pain is not associated with fever.

Primary epiploic appendagitis is inflammation and infarction of the epiploic appendage without an underlying cause.[15] The sonographic features include a small, usually echogenic, noncompressible, ovoid mass, located deep to the abdominal wall in the area of maximal tenderness.[16] Sometimes, a thin, hypoechoic rim may surround the mass.[16]

An important feature that distinguishes epiploic appendagitis from diverticulitis is the absence of thickening of the adjacent bowel wall and the absence of air within the echogenic nodule.[16] Segmental omental infarction (SOI) is caused by thrombosis of omental vessels, resulting in infarction. Ultrasound usually shows a solid, hyperechoic, and noncompressible mass deep to the area of maximal tenderness. The mass may become partly heterogeneous if necrosis from infarction is present; however, abnormal echogenic fat is usually seen around the lesion (**Fig. 8**). The clinical presentations of epiploic appendagitis and SOI are similar and both should be considered in the differential diagnosis of right lower quadrant pain. Both of these entities are self-limiting and resolve spontaneously with conservative management.

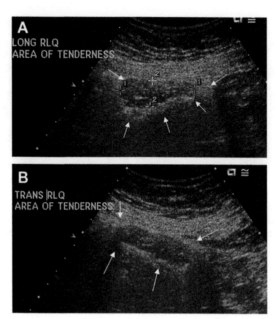

Fig. 8. Epiploic appendagitis. Longitudinal (*A*) and transverse (*B*) ultrasound images through the right lower quadrant show an elongated soft tissue mass seen posterior to the anterior abdominal wall that has heterogeneous texture. A rim of echogenic fat is seen around the lesion (*arrows*). (*Courtesy of* Dr Monser Abu-Yousef.)

COLITIS

Colitis usually shows on ultrasound as a diffuse bowel wall thickening. Thickening of the terminal ileum and the cecum is seen in Crohn's disease. Other findings that may be seen on ultrasound include decreased peristalsis, lack of compressibility, strictures, and hyperemia of the bowel loops. Inflammation and proliferation of the surrounding fat and mesentery leads to noncompressible, echogenic tissues that are seen adjacent to the bowel.[17] This description has been referred to as *creeping fat* and usually occurs at the terminal ileum or cecum.[18–20] The earliest reported finding on ultrasound is presence of small echolucencies within the submucosa. Because all the layers of the bowel wall are thickened, there is loss of the normal striated gut signature. Echogenic foci within the hypoechoic muscularis layer represent ulceration.[17] Complex fluid collections or solid-appearing masses with air may represent abscesses or fistulas around the bowel.

In patients with ulcerative colitis, the rectum is involved first and then the disease extends proximally. Typhlitis is seen as wall thickening predominantly involving the cecum and ascending colon and usually occurs in neutropenic patients with secondary infections. Pseudomembranous colitis causes edema and diffuse wall thickening of the entire colon (**Fig. 9**), usually from *Clostridium difficile* infection in patients on antibiotic therapy. Ischemic colitis usually occurs in the region of splenic flexure and descending colon and is manifested by bowel wall thickening seen in these areas.

BOWEL OBSTRUCTION

Although sonography is not the gold standard for imaging the bowel, occasionally it can help diagnose bowel obstruction. In the cases of suspected bowel obstruction,

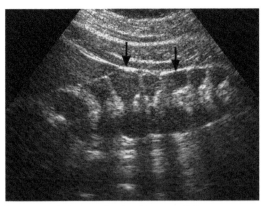

Fig. 9. Pseudomembranous colitis. Longitudinal image of the transverse colon shows thickening of the haustra. (*From* Scoutt LM, Swayers SR, Bokhari J, et al. Ultrasound evaluation of the acute abdomen. Ultrasound Clin 2007;2(3):512; with permission.)

sonographic assessment includes evaluation of caliber differences of various parts of bowel from the stomach to the rectum, exaggerated peristaltic activity, or any findings of intussusception. Occasionally, a large gallstones or a foreign body may be seen at the point of obstruction. The fluid in the dilated bowel serves as contrast medium and distends the bowel loops, making them readily detectable on ultrasound. Peristalsis with a to-and-fro bowel fluid movement may also be noted. Small bowel can be distinguished from colon by the presence of valvulae conniventes and absence of the thick haustral markings of the colon (**Fig. 10**). Sonography has a reported sensitivity of 89% for diagnosing small bowel obstruction.[8,21] Massively distended bowel loops with wall thickening and absent color flow on Doppler ultrasound may indicate bowel infarction. Sonography can also be used to evaluate colonic obstruction and has a reported sensitivity of 88%.[8,21,22] However, CT and plain films remain the preferred imaging modalities for the clinical suspicion of bowel obstruction.

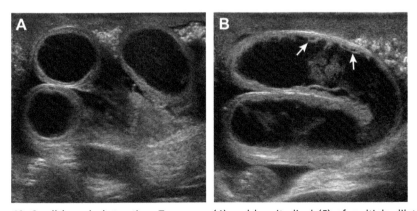

Fig. 10. Small bowel obstruction. Transverse (*A*) and longitudinal (*B*) of multiple dilated loops of small bowel in a patient with distal small bowel obstruction. (*From* Scoutt LM, Sawyers SR, Bokhari J, et al. Ultrasound evaluation of the acute abdomen. Ultrasound Clin 2007;2(3):513; with permission.)

METASTATIC DISEASE

Peritoneal metastatic disease or peritoneal carcinomatosis is defined as metastatic disease to the omentum, peritoneal surface, peritoneal ligaments, or mesentery. The ultrasound findings are better shown in the presence of ascites and include hypoechoic or hyperechoic nodular omental masses seen through the anechoic ascites (**Fig. 11**). Nodular masses may be present on the omentum (omental cake), parietal peritoneum, or serosal surface of the bowel walls. In the absence of ascites, detection of peritoneal implants smaller than 3 mm is difficult. Color Doppler ultrasound may detect vascularity in omental/peritoneal deposits. Thickening of the mesenteric side of the terminal ileum may be seen secondary to desmoplastic reaction.[23]

INGUINAL HERNIAS

Although most inguinal hernias are diagnosed in childhood, they can also present in adulthood as the cause of acute pelvic pain. Ultrasound is considered the primary imaging modality for evaluating inguinal hernias (**Fig. 12**). Color Doppler sonography can be used to differentiate indirect versus direct inguinal hernias.[24] In direct hernias, the hernial defect is seen medial to the inferior epigastric artery, whereas indirect hernias occur through the inguinal canal. Ultrasound is helpful in distinguishing hernias from other groin masses, such as a varicocele, hematoma, or hydrocele.[25]

HYDROCELE

A hydrocele of the canal of Nuck is a rare cause of pain and sometimes can cause inguinal swelling in women. It is embryologically related to an indirect inguinal hernia because it develops in women who have a patent processus vaginalis accompanying the round ligament of the uterus.[26–28] The sonographic appearance is that of a cystic mass with a well-defined echogenic margin (**Fig. 13**). Occasionally, the mass may contain septa or cystic internal structures. Hammond[26] reported a case in which the use of pressure from the ultrasound transducer caused the cyst to be reduced into the peritoneal cavity.

VARICOCELE

A varicocele of the round ligament or labial varicocele is a rare entity that can cause pelvic pain and swelling. The round ligament passes from the pelvis, through the

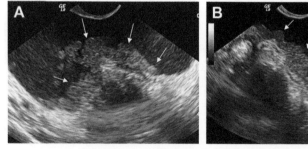

Fig. 11. Peritoneal metastasis. Transverse (*A*) and longitudinal (*B*) ultrasound image through the lower abdomen. Multiple solid irregular masses are seen overlying the peritoneal surface in the lower abdomen (*arrows*). Surrounding ascitic fluid shows internal echoes from hemorrhage.

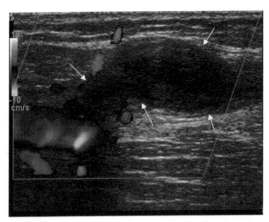

Fig. 12. Right indirect inguinal hernia. A longitudinal color Doppler ultrasound image through the right inguinal region shows an elongated hypoechoic mass within the superficial soft tissues of the inguinal canal (*arrows*). The mass shows a narrow neck (adjacent to the vessel), and the hernial sac mostly contains fat. No flow is noted within the mass.

internal inguinal ring, and along the inguinal canal to the labia majora.[29] The varicocele is usually associated with pregnancy and worsens progressively until delivery. It usually resolves after delivery. Most cases present in the third trimester of pregnancy. Gray-scale sonography shows prominent anechoic tubular channels that reveal venous flow on color Doppler. Augmentation using valsalva maneuvers is helpful because venous flow at rest can be subtle. Sometimes having the patient stand can accentuate the findings (**Fig. 14**A, D).[30]

DUPLICATION CYSTS

Enteric duplication cysts are rare congenital anomalies arising anywhere along the gastrointestinal tract[31] that may cause abdominal or pelvic pain, especially when

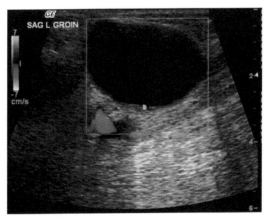

Fig. 13. Hydrocele in the canal of Nuck. An oblique Doppler ultrasound image through the left groin shows an anechoic fluid collection in the left inguinal region. The collection does not show thick walls or color flow.

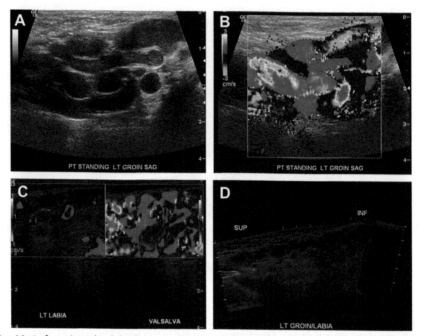

Fig. 14. Left varicocele. (*A*) Ultrasound image through the left groin in standing position that shows multiple anechoic tubular structures. (*B*) Color Doppler image through the same area showing vascular flow in these consistent with varices. (*C*) Dual image through the left labia without (*left*) and with (*right*) Valsalva maneuver. (*D*) Extended-view image through the left groin showing the extent of the varicocele.

complicated by hemorrhage, infection, or torsion. Complicated cysts may present with symptoms similar to appendicitis or ovarian torsion. Duplication cysts are defined by their histologic appearance. Similar to the native gastrointestinal tract, these cysts contain an inner mucosa–submucosa layer surrounded by an outer smooth-muscle layer.[31,32] On imaging, the double wall or "muscular rim" sign has been suggested

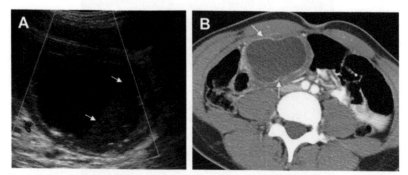

Fig. 15. Complicated duplication cyst with internal hemorrhage. (*A*) Color Doppler image of a thick-walled cystic mass showing no evidence of flow within the walls. Layering debris is noted toward right (*arrows*). (*B*) Axial slice of a contrast-enhanced CT scan through the lower abdomen that shows thick-walled cystic mass with slightly enhanced walls (*arrows*).

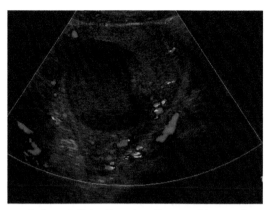

Fig. 16. Infected mesenteric cyst. Color Doppler ultrasound image through the right lower abdomen shows a large thick-walled cystic structure. The fluid shows internal echoes from infection. Increased vascularity is present in the thick walls, suggesting hyperemia.

to be characteristic of duplication cysts.[31,32] The characteristic sonographic appearance includes visualization of an inner hyperechoic rim correlating to the mucosa–submucosa and an outer surrounding hypoechoic layer reflecting muscularis propria.[32–35] Occasionally, these cysts may become infected or show internal hemorrhage (**Figs. 15** and **16**).

SUMMARY

Ultrasound is a valuable noninvasive diagnostic tool for evaluating female patients who present with acute pelvic pain. Although gynecologic conditions constitute most causes of acute pelvic pain, particularly in women of childbearing age; nongynecologic conditions should also be considered. These conditions may be easily overlooked and delay diagnosis. Sometimes ultrasound can help diagnose nongynecologic disorders. Not only is sonography helpful from an imaging standpoint but also one can take advantage of direct patient contact during the examination to correlate the point of maximal tenderness with the underlying imaging findings. Ultrasound should be used as the primary imaging modality in children and pregnant women in whom appendicitis or ureteral calculi is clinically suspected.

REFERENCES

1. Guidry SP, Poole GV. The anatomy of appendicitis. Am Surg 1994;60:68–71.
2. Bongard F, Landers DV, Lewis F. Differential diagnosis of appendicitis and pelvic inflammatory disease. Am J Surg 1985;150:90–6.
3. Puylaert JB. Acute appendicitis: US evaluation using graded compression. Radiology 1986;158:355–60.
4. Jeffrey RB, Jain KA, Nghiem HV. Sonographic diagnosis of acute appendicitis: interpretive pitfalls. Am J Roentgenol 1994;162:55–9.
5. Migraine S, Atri M, Bret PM, et al. Spontaneously resolving acute appendicitis: clinical and sonographic documentation. Radiology 1997;205:55–8.
6. Bau A, Atri M. Acute female pelvic pain: ultrasound evaluation. Semin Ultrasound CT MR 2000;2(1):78–93.

7. Angle R, Ackerman S, Irshad A. Practical imaging of acute pelvic pain in premenopausal women. Contemp Diagn Radiol 2010;33(1):1–6.
8. Kuzmich S, Howlett D, Andi A. Transabdominal sonography in assessment of the bowel in adults. Am J Roentgenol 2009;192:197–212.
9. Hollerweger A, Rettenbacher T, Macheiner P, et al. Sigmoid diverticulitis: value of transrectal sonography in addition to transabdominal sonography. Am J Roentgenol 2000;175:1155–60.
10. Hollerweger A. Colonic diseases: the value of US examination. Eur J Radiol 2007; 64:239–49.
11. Yilmaz S, Sindel T, Arslan G, et al. Renal colic: comparison of spiral CT, US and IVU in the detection of ureteral calculi. Eur Radiol 1998;8:212–7.
12. Patlas M, Farkas A, Fisher D, et al. Ultrasound vs CT for the detection of ureteric stones in patients with renal colic. Br J Radiol 2001;74:901–4.
13. Platt JF. Doppler ultrasound of the kidney. Semin Ultrasound CT MR 1997;18: 22–32.
14. Simanovsky N, Hiller N. Importance of sonographic detection in enlarged abdominal lymph nodes in children. J Ultrasound Med 2007;26:581–4.
15. McClure M, Khalili K, Sarrazin J, et al. Radiological features of epiploic appendagitis and segmental omental infarction. Clin Radiol 2001;56:819–27.
16. Rioux M, Lanigs P. Primary epiploic appendagitis: clinical, US, and CT findings in 14 cases. Radiology 1994;191:523–6.
17. Scoutt L, Sawyers S, Bokhari J, et al. Ultrasound evaluation of the acute abdomen. Ultrasound Clin 2007;2(3):493–523.
18. Puylaert JB. Ultrasonography of the acute abdomen: gastrointestinal conditions. Radiol Clin North Am 2003;41:1227–42.
19. Sarrazin J, Wilson S. Manifestations of Crohn's disease at US. Radiographics 1996;84:385–8.
20. Maconi G, Radice E, Greco A, et al. Bowel ultrasound in Crohn's disease. Best Pract Res Clin Gastroenterol 2006;20:93–112.
21. Schmutz G, Benko A, Fournier L, et al. Small bowel obstruction: role and contribution of sonography. Eur Radiol 1997;7:1054–8.
22. Lim JH, Yt Ko, Lee DH, et al. Determining the site and causes of colonic obstruction with sonography. Am J Roentgenol 1994;163:1113–7.
23. Lolge S. Peritoneal carcinomatosis. In: Ahuja A, editor. Diagnostic imaging: ultrasound. 1st edition. Salt Lake City (UT): Amirsys; 2007. p. 14–7.
24. Atri M, Migraine S, Nazari A, et al. Impact of endovaginal sonography on the evaluation of patients with clinical diagnosis of diverticulitis. Radiology 1997; 205:193.
25. Korenkov M, Paul A, Troidl H. Color duplex sonography: diagnostic tool in the differentiation of inguinal hernias. J Ultrasound Med 1999;18(8):565–8.
26. Hammond I. Letter to the editor: cyst of the canal of Nuck. J Ultrasound Med 2007;26:147.
27. Stickel WH, Manner M. Female hydrocele: sonographic appearance of a rare and little known disorder. J Ultrasound Med 2004;23:429–32.
28. Yigit H, Tuncbilek I, Fitoz S, et al. Cyst of the canal of Nuck with demonstration of the proximal canal: the role of the compression technique in sonographic diagnosis. J Ultrasound Med 2006;25:123–5.
29. Murphy IG, Heffernan EJ, Gibney RG, et al. Groin mass in pregnancy. Br J Radiol 2007;80:588–9.
30. Nguyen Q, Gruenewald M. Doppler sonography in the diagnosis of round ligament varicosities during pregnancy. J Clin Ultrasound 2008;36(3):177–9.

31. Cheng G, Soboleski D, Daneman A, et al. Sonographic pitfalls in the diagnosis of enteric duplication cysts. Am J Roentgenol 2005;184:521–5.
32. Ros PR, Olmsted WW, Moser RP, et al. Mesenteric and omental cysts: histologic classification with imaging correlation. Radiology 1987;164:327–32.
33. Segal SR, Sherman NH, Rosenberg HK, et al. Ultrasonographic features of gastrointestinal duplications. J Ultrasound Med 1994;13:863–70.
34. Kangarloo H, Sample WR, Hansen G, et al. Ultrasonic evaluation of abdominal gastrointestinal tract duplication in children. Radiology 1979;131:191–4.
35. Moccia W, Astacio J, Kauge J, et al. Ultrasonographic demonstration of gastric duplication in infancy. Pediatr Radiol 1981;11:2–54.

Ultrasound Evaluation of Gynecologic Causes of Pelvic Pain

Lawrence A. Cicchiello, MD[a],*, Ulrike M. Hamper, MD, MBA[b],
Leslie M. Scoutt, MD[c]

KEYWORDS

• Pelvic pain • Ultrasound • Gynecologic • Obstetric

Acute pelvic pain, defined as noncyclic pain lasting for less than 3 months, is a common presenting symptom of premenopausal women in an emergency department or physician's office. Acute pelvic pain is a nonspecific symptom and there is a broad range of gynecologic and nongynecologic causes, including gastrointestinal, urologic, and musculoskeletal etiologies. Acute pelvic pain is often associated with other nonspecific signs and symptoms, including nausea, vomiting, and leukocytosis. Hence, imaging is frequently required to narrow the differential diagnosis, and endovaginal ultrasound (EVUS) is the most widely accepted initial imaging modality of choice if there is high clinical suspicion for obstetric or gynecologic etiologies.[1]

Chronic pelvic pain is defined as noncyclic pain lasting longer than 6 months. Approximately 14% of women in the United States report symptoms of chronic pelvic pain, but the cause is often undiagnosed.[2,3] The most common gynecologic causes of chronic pelvic pain include adenomyosis, endometriosis, leiomyomas, adhesions, and pelvic congestion syndrome.[4] Ultrasound (US) is most helpful in the diagnosis of leiomyomas, adenomyosis, and endometriosis. This article reviews the role of US in the evaluation of gynecologic causes of acute and chronic pelvic pain.

ACUTE PELVIC PAIN

Gynecologic causes of acute pelvic pain can be further categorized into obstetric and nonobstetric causes. Therefore, the first step in the evaluation of a premenopausal

A version of this article was previously published in *Ultrasound Clinics* 5:2.
[a] Department of Diagnostic Radiology, Yale University School of Medicine, 333 Cedar Street, PO Box 208042, New Haven, CT 06520-8042, USA
[b] Division of Ultrasound, Department of Diagnostic Radiology, The Johns Hopkins Medical Institutes, 600 North Wolfe Street, Baltimore, MD 21287, USA
[c] Ultrasound Service, Department of Diagnostic Radiology, Yale University School of Medicine, 333 Cedar Street, PO Box 208042, New Haven, CT 06520-8042, USA
* Corresponding author. Department of Diagnostic Radiology, Yale-New Haven Hospital, 20 York Street, New Haven, CT 06511.
E-mail address: lcicchiello@gmail.com

Obstet Gynecol Clin N Am 38 (2011) 85–114
doi:10.1016/j.ogc.2011.02.005
0889-8545/11/$ – see front matter © 2011 Elsevier Inc. All rights reserved.

woman with acute pelvic pain is to establish if the patient is pregnant, with a β–human chorionic gonadotropion (hCG) level. Common gynecologic causes of pelvic pain in nonpregnant patients include large ovarian cysts, ruptured or hemorrhagic cysts, pelvic inflammatory disease (PID), ovarian or adnexal torsion, and malpositioned intrauterine devices (IUDs). Because many of these conditions may also occur during pregnancy, they should also be considered in pregnant patients with pelvic pain. Common gynecologic causes of pelvic pain associated with pregnancy include hemorrhagic corpus luteums (CL), spontaneous abortion (SAB), ectopic pregnancy (EP), subchorionic hemorrhage, pain associated with ovarian hyperstimulation syndrome (OHSS), and degenerated fibroids. Postpartum causes of pelvic pain include endometritis, retained products of conception (RPOCs), ovarian vein thrombophlebitis, and rupture of the uterus.[5]

ACUTE PELVIC PAIN IN NONPREGNANT PATIENTS
Simple Ovarian Cysts

Most ovarian follicles measure less than 1 cm in diameter. The dominant follicle typically measures less than 2.5 cm at the time of ovulation. A follicle that fails to release an oocyte or does not regress can enlarge into a follicular cyst and accounts for the vast majority of simple ovarian cystic structures. The term, *follicular cyst*, is reserved for lesions measuring greater than 3 cm, but these lesions can often grow larger, especially during pregnancy. Small ovarian cysts are common but usually asymptomatic and have been reported in up to 7% of asymptomatic premenopausal women.[6] Large or enlarging ovarian cysts, however, can be a source of pelvic pain, and cysts larger than 5 cm are believed to predispose to ovarian torsion. Sonographically, follicular cysts appear as unilocular anechoic intraovarian or exophytic ovarian masses with thin, imperceptible walls and posterior acoustic enhancement. When follicular cysts become large, it may be difficult to appreciate the adjacent ovarian parenchyma, which may be compressed or hidden from view (**Fig. 1**). In premenopausal women, the risk of malignancy in a simple ovarian cyst is low.[7] The current recommendation by the Society of Radiologists in Ultrasound is that asymptomatic simple ovarian cysts

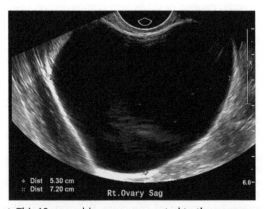

Fig. 1. Follicular cyst. This 19-year-old woman presented to the emergency department with acute pelvic pain. EVUS reveals a large right adnexal anechoic cystic structure (*calipers*) in the region of the patient's pain consistent with a follicular cyst. The wall is smooth and there is posterior wall enhancement. The origin of the pain is not certain in this patient and could be due to mass effect, stretching of the capsule of the cyst or ovary, torquing of the ovarian pedicle, or leakage.

larger than 7 cm in premenopausal women should be referred for evaluation with MRI to ensure that mural nodularity is not missed due to sampling error with US.[8] Asymptomatic simple cysts greater than 5 cm but less than 7 cm in diameter are amenable to yearly follow-up with US. Follow-up is not necessary for asymptomatic simple cysts less than or equal to 5 cm in diameter in the reproductive age group.[8]

Ruptured or Hemorrhagic Ovarian Cysts

The most common gynecologic cause of acute pelvic pain in nonpregnant, afebrile premenopausal women presenting to an emergency department is a ruptured or hemorrhagic ovarian cyst. Ruptured or hemorrhagic ovarian cysts typically present with acute-onset, severe, but self-limited, unilateral pelvic pain. Patients are most commonly afebrile with a normal white blood cell count. If the cyst is leaking, rebound tenderness may be present. If there is a large amount of intra-abdominal bleeding, patients may be hypotensive or present with syncope. A ruptured ovarian cyst may be a diagnosis of exclusion on US examination because the ovary may appear completely normal if the cyst has completely ruptured and the fluid resorbed or dispersed throughout the peritoneal cavity. A leaking ovarian cyst may have a crenated appearance, however, containing low-level echoes or clot. Adjacent free fluid may be noted (**Fig. 2**).[9] On US, hemoperitoneum, which is most commonly found in the cul-de-sac, is diagnosed by the presence of free intraperitoneal fluid containing low-level echoes. Free intraperitoneal fluid often has a triangular or pointed configuration as it interdigitates between loops of bowel and pelvic structures. If there is a large amount of bleeding, heterogeneous masses of clot may be observed within the fluid or surrounding the uterus and ovary (**Fig. 3**). Clot can be distinguished from adjacent bowel by the lack of vascularity on Doppler interrogation and absence of peristalsis. Bowel also has a tubular configuration. If there is a substantial amount of bleeding, hemoperitoneum extends from the pelvis into the upper abdomen. Hence, the hepatorenal recess, or Morison pouch, as well as the left upper quadrant should be evaluated transabdominally for the presence of blood (see **Fig. 2**).[10] This constellation of findings can mimic a ruptured EP, and a β-hCG level should be obtained in any premenopausal women presenting with acute pelvic pain, hemoperitoneum, or syncope.[11] The US findings of hemoperitoneum are nonspecific, however, and echoes within fluid can also be caused by debris or infection.

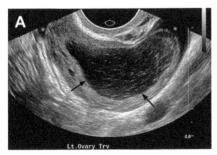 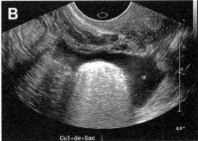

Fig. 2. Leaking hemorrhagic ovarian cyst. This 18-year-old woman presented to the emergency department with acute, left-sided, pelvic pain. (*A*) Transverse EVUS image of the left ovary reveals a collapsing, crenated hemorrhagic left ovarian cyst (*arrows*). Note adjacent free fluid (*asterisk*) and fine reticular stranding within the cyst consistent with hemorrhage. (*B*) Image of the cul-de-sac reveals free fluid (*asterisk*) containing low-level echoes consistent with hemoperitoneum.

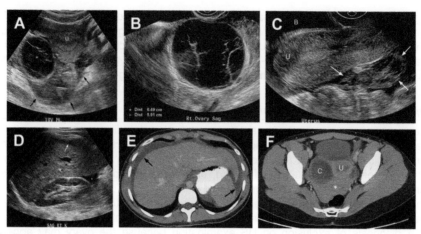

Fig. 3. Ruptured hemorrhagic ovarian cyst. This 33-year-old woman presented to the emergency department with syncope after abrupt onset of right-sided pelvic pain. (*A*) Transverse transabdominal image of the pelvis reveals a large right adnexal cystic structure (*asterisk*) with internal septations. Note large amount of adjacent clot and complex free fluid consistent with hemoperitoneum (*arrows*). The uterus (U) has an arcuate configuration. (*B*) EVUS image reveals fine, irregular septations within the cyst (*calipers*) consistent with fibrin stranding. (*C*) Sagittal midline EVUS image reveals free fluid and clotted blood (*arrows*) in the cul-de-sac posterior to the uterus (U). Note small amount of free fluid superior to the uterine fundus underneath the bladder (B). (*D*) Transabdominal US image of the right upper quadrant reveals free fluid (*asterisk*) in Morison pouch and also between the liver and the diaphragm (*arrow*). The presence of clotted blood in the cul-de-sac as well as fluid in the right upper quadrant suggests that there has been a large amount of bleeding. (*E*) CT scan of the upper abdomen reveals fluid around the liver and spleen (*arrows*). (*F*) CT scan of the pelvis reveals dense fluid (*asterisk*) in the cul-de-sac consistent with hemorrhage. Note hemorrhagic right ovarian cyst (C) and uterus (U) posterior to the bladder.

The sonographic appearance of hemorrhagic cysts is variable depending on when, in the evolution of the hemorrhage, patients are imaged. Acutely, a hemorrhagic cyst on US examination demonstrates a pattern of diffuse, low-level, internal echoes; no internal vascularity; a thin wall; and increased through transmission. As the red blood cells lyse and fibrin strands form within the hemorrhagic cyst, a lace-like or fishnet reticular pattern of internal echoes is observed (**Fig. 4**). These strands should be thin, smooth, and avascular. Over time, echogenic thrombus coalesces within the cyst, forming a heterogenous avascular mass with retractile (angular or concave) margins (**Fig. 5**). Clot within a hemorrhagic cyst is usually dependent but can become adherent to the cyst wall as it evolves. Intraluminal clot can occasionally have a more rounded configuration and thereby mimic the US appearance of a mural nodule within a cystic ovarian neoplasm.[12] Although lack of vascularity on Doppler interrogation within a focal echogenic area in an ovarian cyst favors the diagnosis of hemorrhagic clot, Doppler US is not 100% sensitive for the depiction of tumor vascularity. Therefore, follow-up imaging in 6 to 8 weeks in such cases is recommended. Clots resolve or change in that time frame.[12] If vascularity develops or if the area increases in size or even stays the same, a tumor nodule should be strongly suspected.

Pelvic Inflammatory Disease

Pelvic inflammatory disease (PID) includes a spectrum of sexually transmitted infections of the cervix, uterus, fallopian tubes, and ovaries. The classic clinical symptoms

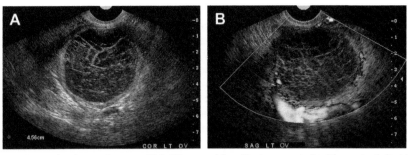

Fig. 4. Hemorrhagic ovarian cyst. This 24-year-old patient presented with acute, left-sided, pelvic pain. (*A*) EVUS of the left ovary reveals a 4.56-cm cystic mass (*calipers*) demonstrating a reticular lace-like pattern of internal echoes and strand-like septations. (*B*) Power Doppler EVUS image reveals a small amount of blood flow in the wall of the cyst but no evidence of internal vascularity.

of acute PID include pelvic pain, cervical motion tenderness, vaginal discharge, fever, and leukocytosis. The severity of the pain is variable, ranging from mild pelvic discomfort to severe bilateral lower quadrant pain. Most cases are caused by *Chlamydia trachomatis* or *Neisseria gonorrhoeae*, but coinfection with other bacteria is common.[13] PID is an ascending infection beginning as cervicitis, ultimately spreading upwards through the genital tract to involve first the endometrium (endometritis) and then the fallopian tubes (salpingitis). As the purulent material spills out into the peritoneal cavity from the fimbriated ends of the fallopian tubes, it typically coats the serosal surface of the uterus causing a serositis and eventually engulfs the adjacent ovary forming a tubo-ovarian abscess (TOA). PID is most commonly a bilateral process involving both adnexa, although sometimes to different degrees. Less commonly, TOAs can be the result of direct spread of infection to the adnexa from intra-abdominal infections, usually from the bowel, such as appendicitis or diverticulitis. Although endometritis most often occurs in the setting of PID, endometritis may also occur post partum or after instrumentation.

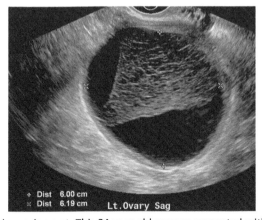

Fig. 5. Hemorrhagic ovarian cyst. This 34-year-old woman presented with acute, left-sided, pelvic pain for 2 days. EVUS reveals a cystic structure (*calipers*) in the left adnexa. Note moth-eaten appearance of the central area of internal echoes, which has straight/concave margins consistent with retractile clot. Doppler interrogation (not shown) revealed no internal vascularity.

Because the symptoms of PID are frequently nonspecific, endovaginal sonography can be a useful adjunct to the clinical presentation in the diagnosis of PID. Although EVUS is most sensitive for detecting ovarian and tubal involvement of disease, with sensitivity of 90% and 93%, respectively, it is less sensitive for the detection of cervical or uterine involvement.[14] In early acute PID, when only the cervix is involved, US examination is typically normal, and the diagnosis of cervicitis is usually made by visual inspection and culture. Sonographic findings of endometritis include the presence of fluid or gas within the endometrial canal, heterogeneous thickening of the endometrial stripe, and indistinctness of the endometrial stripe. Echogenic foci with distal shadowing may indicate the presence of air within the infected debris in the endometrial cavity (**Fig. 6**). Doppler interrogation may demonstrate increased, low-resistance vascularity. Inflammation of the fallopian tubes manifests as thickening of the tube with increased vascularity. Hydrosalpinx, or a dilated, fluid-filled fallopian tube, can develop secondary to obstruction from pelvic adhesions or post inflammatory scarring and appears sonographically as a tubular anechoic adnexal structure, often U- or S-shaped. It is common for a dilated tube to fold on itself. When this occurs, the inner walls of the tube along the fold compress together creating the appearance of an incomplete septation. The dilated tube can have a cogwheel appearance on transverse images with multiple tiny mural protrusions representing the inflamed folded/redundant tubal mucosa. In patients with chronic salpingitis, the tube may demonstrate a beads-on-a-string appearance.[15] The presence of low-level echoes or layering with a fluid-debris level in a dilated, fluid-filled tube suggests the diagnosis of pyosalpinx (**Fig. 7**). The presence of a thin hypoechoic rim, likely representing fluid and purulent material, surrounding the uterus suggests inflammation of the serosal surface of the uterus (uterine serositis). Finally, when the infection involves the fallopian tube and ovary, a tubo-ovarian complex or abscess develops, which manifests sonographically as a complex thick-walled, multilocular cystic collection in the adnexa. Typically, internal echoes or multiple fluid-fluid levels are observed within the locules (**Fig. 8**). The walls and septations of TOAs are usually hypervascular with a low-resistance arterial waveform pattern. Acute TOAs are usually bilateral and tender on US examination. TOA is used to describe lesions with complete breakdown

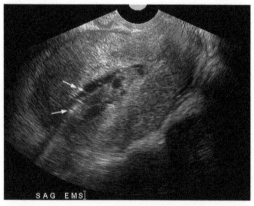

Fig. 6. Endometritis. This 23-year-old woman presented with pelvic pain, fever, and purulent discharge. Sagittal EVUS images of the uterus demonstrate a thick, heterogeneous, endometrial stripe consistent with the presence of debris, hemorrhage, or purulent material. The outer margins of the endometrial stripe are indistinct. Echogenic areas (*arrows*) with posterior shadowing and ring-down artifact are consistent with the presence of air.

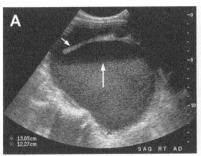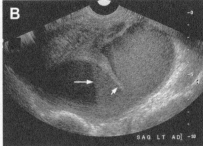

Fig. 7. Pyosalpinx. (*A, B*) EVUS images of the left adnexa in this 19-year-old woman with pelvic pain and fever demonstrate a dilated tubular structure (*calipers* in [*A*]) filled with debris/purulent material consistent with a pyosalpinx. Note fluid/fluid layering (*long arrow*) and incomplete septation (*short arrow*) where the tube folds on itself. Note that the fimbriated end of the tube is larger than the more medial portion.

of tubal and ovarian architecture.[14–16] If an ovarian capsule or some ovarian tissue is preserved, the term, *tubo-ovarian complex*, is used. Tubo-ovarian complexes usually respond better to antibiotic therapy than TOAs. Purulent fluid, with increased echogenicity and debris, can be seen in the cul-de-sac. Increased echogenicity of the pelvic fat also can be seen occasionally (**Fig. 9**) and is the sonographic correlate of fat stranding commonly seen on CT in patients with inflammatory disorders.[16]

Pelvic abscesses may occur after surgery or trauma or may develop secondary to bowel pathology. Patients most often present with acute pain, fever, and leukocytosis. Rebound tenderness may be present. The degree of pain may be variable and the presenting symptoms are nonspecific. Although CT is generally considered the imaging modality of choice in women with suspected pelvic abscess, US is an alternative imaging choice in pregnant or younger patients because it avoids the risk of radiation exposure. In addition, abscesses may be found when a patient is imaged with US for other suspected pathology.

On US, pelvic abscesses appear as complex, often irregularly marginated, multilocular fluid collections containing low-level echoes (**Fig. 10**). The internal echogenicity may range from hypoechoic to quite echogenic if air or subacute bleeding is present.

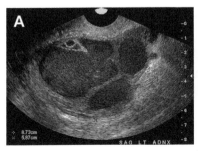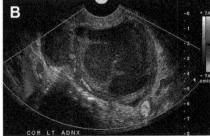

Fig. 8. Tubo-ovarian abscess. This 23-year-old woman presented with pelvic pain, fever, and purulent vaginal discharge. (*A*) Sagittal EVUS image of the left adnexal reveals a complex multilocular cystic mass (*calipers*) with thick irregular septations and low-level echoes within the cystic components consistent with debris, pus, or hemorrhage. (*B*) Color Doppler image demonstrating vascularity in the wall of the TOA. This mass was tender on physical examination.

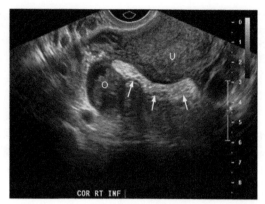

Fig. 9. Echogenic pelvic fat. Note increased echogenicity in the pelvic fat (*arrows*) between the uterus (U) and the right ovary (O) in this 23-year-old woman with PID. Increased echogenicity in the pelvic fat is a nonspecific finding indicative of inflammation or infection and may be seen on US examination in patients with Crohn disease, ulcerative colitis, diverticulitis, and appendicitis.

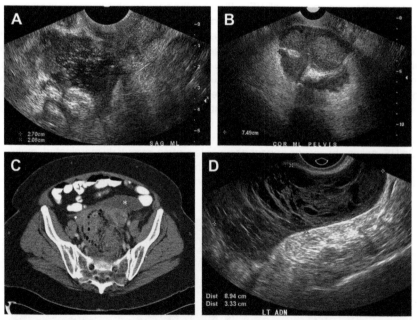

Fig. 10. Pelvic abscess. (*A*) Sagittal EVUS images in a patient status–post hysterectomy who presents with pelvic pain and fever. Note fluid collection (*calipers*) containing debris/purulent material in the midline superior to the vaginal cuff. (*B*) This second patient also presented with pelvic pain and fever. EVUS revealed a complex, irregular cystic mass (*calipers*) in the region of the patient's pain. (*C*) CT scan demonstrates diverticular abscess containing air and fluid. Note free intraperitoneal air and adjacent free fluid (*asterisk*) as well as many diverticula arising from the sigmoid colon. (*D*) In this third patient with a pelvic abscess status–post hysterectomy, note fluid collection (*calipers*) with many fine reticular septations in the left adnexa.

The walls may be vascular with a low-resistance arterial waveform pattern. Adjacent purulent fluid containing low-level echoes may be noted. Pelvic hematomas may be indistinguishable (**Fig. 11**) and may also present with acute pelvic pain. Aspiration may be required to exclude superinfection although the wall of an abscess is typically more echogenic and vascular than the wall of a hematoma.

Ovarian Torsion

Ovarian torsion accounts for approximately 3% of all gynecologic emergencies.[17] It is defined as partial or complete twisting of the ovary or fallopian tube around its vascular pedicle. Torsion of the vascular pedicle initially results in lymphatic and venous obstruction and, if not relieved, eventually progresses to compromise arterial flow. In up to 67% of cases, the ovary and fallopian tube are twisted together resulting in adnexal torsion.[18] The right adnexa is more commonly involved.[17] Adnexal torsion is a surgical emergency and timely diagnosis and intervention are required to preserve vascularity and prevent ovarian necrosis. The chance of salvaging viable ovarian tissue markedly decreases if symptoms have persisted for longer than 48 hours.[19] Risk factors for ovarian torsion include the presence of an ipsilateral adnexal mass, pregnancy, ovulation induction, prior tubal ligation, and hypermobility of adnexal structures.[17,18,20–22] An ipsilateral adnexal mass greater than 5 cm is the most common risk factor and is reported to be present in 22% to 73% of cases.[17,18,21,22] Dermoids are reportedly the most commonly associated lesion, present in up to 20% of cases.[18] Malignant lesions are less likely than benign lesions to cause adnexal torsion, with 1 series reporting less than 1% of cases involving a malignant lesion.[20] Larger masses (>10 cm) are less likely to undergo torsion probably due to the larger weight as well as compression or fixation in place by adjacent pelvic structures. Although adnexal torsion occurs most commonly in women of reproductive age, ovarian torsion is reported in all age groups, including in utero. Hypermobility of adnexal structures is believed to be the most common predisposing risk factor in children and adolescents. Isolated torsion of the fallopian tube is most common in the adolescent age group.

Classically, patients with adnexal torsion are of reproductive age and present with acute onset of excruciating pelvic pain associated with nausea, vomiting, and adnexal

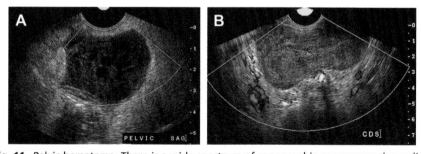

Fig. 11. Pelvic hematoma. There is a wide spectrum of sonographic appearance depending on the length of time since the hemorrhage occurred. The sonographic findings overlap with those of pelvic abscess and, depending on the clinical presentation, aspiration may be required to exclude superinfection of a hematoma. (*A*) Note avascular hypoechoic collection with coalescent anechoic spaces on this color Doppler image. The US appearance is reminiscent of a hemorrhagic cyst. Note triangular outer margins as the hematoma collects between loops of the bowel. (*B*) In this second patient, the hematoma is more echogenic with well-defined smooth margins similar to the US appearance of clotted blood. Power Doppler interrogation revealed no evidence of blood flow.

tenderness. The greater the pain, the higher the concern for ovarian torsion. In more than half of all patients with adnexal torsion, however, the pelvic pain is reported as mild or intermittent.[20–22] A pelvic or abdominal mass is a common presentation of adnexal torsion in children and adolescents. Although there is usually no accompanying fever or leukocytosis, occasionally a mildly elevated white blood cell count can be found. Because of the often confusing clinical picture and overlap of clinical presentation with other causes of pelvic pain, including gastrointestinal pathology and renal colic, a CT scan is often the first imaging study performed. If ovarian torsion is clinically suspected, however, EVUS should be the initial imaging modality of choice.

The sonographic findings of ovarian torsion are variable and often depend on the degree of twisting, the tightness of the torquing, the duration of the torsion, whether or not the fallopian tube has also undergone torsion, and whether or not the torsion is intermittent.[23] The ovarian pedicle may have multiple geometric twists, but if there is no pressure to pull the twisted vessels tight, the blood supply may not be compromised. The classic gray-scale US features of ovarian torsion are enlargement of the ovary, which is often found in a midline position; heterogeneity of the central stroma with echogenic areas representing hemorrhage and hypoechoic areas indicative of edema; and peripheral displacement of the ovarian follicles (**Fig. 12**).[19,23] These findings are not always seen, especially if the duration of symptoms has been long (**Fig. 13**). A longstanding infarcted ovary may have a more complex or amorphous morphologic appearance with cystic degeneration. In almost all cases of ovarian torsion, the ovary is tender. An underlying ovarian mass is often identified (**Fig. 14**). A thickened, swollen tubular structure between the ovary and uterus representing the twisted vascular pedicle may be seen. In cross section, this twisted vascular pedicle demonstrates a target appearance on gray-scale imaging with alternating hyperechoic and hypoechoic bands/circles.[24] On color Doppler, the twisted vessels within the vascular pedicle are described as a whirlpool sign.[25] Adjacent free fluid may be noted. If the fallopian tube alone has undergone torsion, a hydrosalpinx with beaking or angular tapering of the twisted end may be observed.

Spectral Doppler findings in women with adnexal torsion are variable.[26–28] Absence of arterial flow is a highly specific finding for ovarian torsion with a positive predictive value of 94% in 1 study.[26] This is a late finding of ovarian torsion, however, and often indicates that the ovary is not viable. Abnormal vascularity is frequently seen, including decreased or absent diastolic flow and absent venous flow.[28] Completely normal arterial and venous ovarian flow has been described, however, in surgically proven cases of ovarian torsion (see **Figs. 12** and **13**). Therefore, if the gray-scale appearance is suggestive of ovarian torsion, a normal Doppler examination does not exclude the diagnosis. One series reported normal Doppler US findings in up to 60% of cases.[27] This may be due to varying degrees of twisting and tightening of the twists, the intermittent nature of adnexal torsion, and the dual blood supply to the ovary from the ovarian and uterine arteries.

To accurately use Doppler interrogation to evaluate for arterial flow in suspected cases of adnexal torsion, the Doppler settings must be optimized for detection of low velocity flow. This includes setting the color/spectral gain as high as possible without causing noise and motion artifact. The color scale and pulse repetition frequency should be decreased and the wall filter should also be set to low.[29] A small straight color box should be used and attention should be focused on the area between the ovary and uterus near the uterine fundus to search for the twisted pedicle.

Pitfalls in sonographic diagnosis of ovarian torsion include the coexistence of an underlying complex ovarian mass, which can obscure visualization of the normal

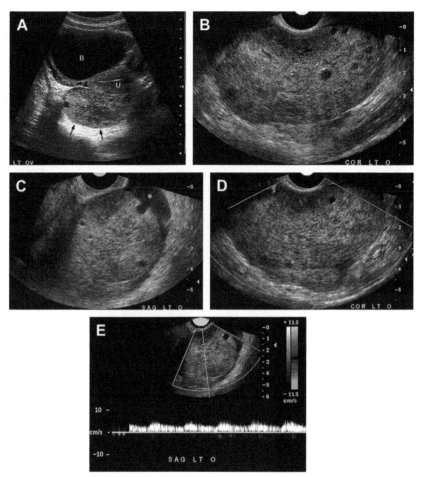

Fig. 12. Ovarian torsion. This 33-year-old woman presented with intermittent left pelvic pain. (*A*) Transabdominal image reveals a markedly enlarged left ovary (*arrows*) located midline in the cul-de-sac posterior to the uterus (U) and bladder (B). (*B, C*) EVUS gray-scale images show to better advantage the heterogenous central ovarian stroma and peripheral displacement of small follicles in the enlarged left ovary. No underlying mass is seen. (*C*) Note small amount of adjacent free fluid (*asterisk*). (*D*) Color Doppler image demonstrates venous and arterial flow (*red and blue*). (*E*) Spectral Doppler tracing reveals a normal arterial waveform. The presence of normal arterial and venous flow does not exclude the diagnosis of ovarian torsion.

ovarian architecture. For example, acoustic attenuation from calcifications or fat in a dermoid cyst can limit evaluation of the remainder of the ovary. In general, if a dermoid is tender on examination, there must be concern for torsion or rupture (see **Fig. 14**). Also, in the presence of OHSS, the ovary becomes enlarged and the ovarian architecture is markedly distorted, making the diagnosis of ovarian torsion difficult.

Malpositon of Intrauterine Devices

IUDs should be positioned in the center of the endometrial cavity in the uterine fundus. Localization of an IUD is most readily accomplished with EVUS. Penetration of the

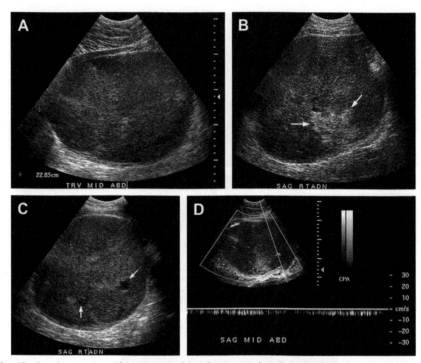

Fig. 13. Ovarian torsion. This 16-year-old girl presented with a large pelvic mass. (*A*) Transabdominal image reveals a largely homogeneous 22.8-cm pelvic mass (*calipers*). (*B*) Careful inspection reveals a geographic echogenic area (*arrows*) consistent with hemorrhagic infarction and (*C*) several small cysts (*arrows*), which confirm that this mass is an enlarged ovary. (*D*) Despite the presence of venous flow on this spectral and power Doppler image, the ovary was infarcted at surgery, which also revealed a large underlying fibrothecoma, which was not prospectively identified on US examination.

myometrium or perforation of the uterus is a rare complication of IUDs (**Figs. 15** and **16**). Such patients most often present with pelvic pain or loss of visualization of the string within the endocervical canal. Occasionally, penetration of the myometrium may be an incidental finding. Recent literature suggests that 3-D US is more accurate and sensitive than EVUS alone for identifying myometrial penetration of IUDs.[30]

ACUTE PELVIC PAIN ASSOCIATED WITH PREGNANCY
Corpus Luteum

A corpus luteum is the remnant of a mature ovarian follicle after ovulation and is frequently seen during the secretory phase of the menstrual cycle. If a patient becomes pregnant, the CL secretes progesterone, which serves to maintain the pregnancy until the placenta forms. Although usually asymptomatic, leaking from or hemorrhage into the CL can cause unilateral pelvic pain or tenderness. Rarely, clinically significant hemoperitoneum can result from rupture of a CL (see **Fig. 3**). A normal CL has a variety of sonographic appearances. Most commonly on US, the CL appears as a round anechoic intraovarian or exophytic ovarian cystic mass with a homogeneous thick moderately echogenic wall, which may be highly vascular with a low-resistance arterial waveform (**Fig. 17**).[31] CLs are usually under 3 cm in size.

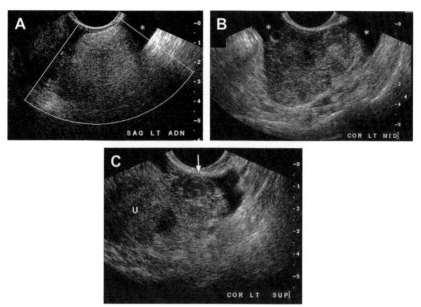

Fig. 14. Torsion of an ovarian dermoid. This 24-year-old woman presented with acute, left-sided, pelvic pain. (*A*) EVUS color Doppler image of the left adnexa reveals a homogeneously echogenic left adnexal mass with posterior attenuation in the region of the patient's pain. Findings are consistent with a dermoid. No color flow is identified. Because ovarian dermoids are primarily cystic, however, blood flow is rarely seen on color Doppler imaging. Tenderness on examination and adjacent free fluid (*asterisk*) are clues to the possibility of torsion or rupture which can also cause pelvic pain. In a patient with a painful dermoid, every attempt should be made to look for the pedicle between the dermoid and the uterus as well as the adjacent ovarian parenchyma because of the clinical concern for torsion. (*B*) EVUS image slightly more superior and midline reveals the adjacent ovary, which is enlarged with heterogeneity of the central stroma. Note peripheral displacement of small follicles and adjacent free fluid (*asterisk*), findings suggestive of ovarian torsion. (*C*) EVUS image more superiorly reveals the target sign (*arrow*) in a transverse plane through the swollen and twisted vascular pedicle between the ovary/dermoid below (not shown) and the uterus (U) confirming the diagnosis of torsion.

Hemorrhage into a CL can create a sonographic pattern of internal echoes similar to a hemorrhagic follicular cyst (see **Figs. 4** and **5**) and rupture of the cyst can result in hemorrhage or clot surrounding the ovary or within the peritoneal cavity (see **Figs. 2** and **3**). Occasionally the CL has a diffusely homogeneous echotexture similar in echogenicity to the ovarian stroma and mimics the US appearance of a solid ovarian mass. Color Doppler interrogation may demonstrate marked vascularity in the wall, thereby separating the CL from the surrounding ovarian parenchyma. These findings are nonspecific, however, and in pregnant patients an exophytic CL may be difficult to differentiate from an EP. Great care must be taken to confirm the presence of an intrauterine pregnancy (IUP). Correlation with serum β-hCG levels may also be helpful in these cases.

Subchorionic Hemorrhage

Subchorionic hemorrhage is defined as separation of the chorion and the endometrial lining by blood, which collects within the subchorionic space. Small subchorionic

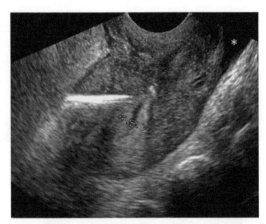

Fig. 15. Malposition of an IUD. This 26-year-old woman presented with pain and vaginal bleeding 2 years status–post placement of an IUD. Sagittal endovaginal image of the uterus reveals a small amount of fluid between the anterior and posterior layers of the endometrium (*calipers*). The IUD, an echogenic linear structure with distal shadowing, has penetrated the anterior myometrial wall and extends beyond the serosal surface of the uterus. Note small amount of free fluid (*asterisk*) in the cul-de-sac.

hemorrhages are common and usually asymptomatic. Large collections may present with vaginal bleeding or abdominal pain or cramping. The echogenicity of a subchorionic hemorrhage varies over time. Acute hemorrhage typically appears more echogenic whereas subacute to chronic hemorrhages can appear hypoechoic **(Fig. 18)**.[32] The outcome of subchorionic hemorrhage is likely related to the size of the collection, maternal age, gestational age, and the presence or absence of pain.[32–34]

Spontaneous Abortion

SAB is defined as pregnancy loss before 20 weeks gestational age, but the majority of SABs occur during the first 16 weeks. Causes of SAB include genetic or fetal causes, structural uterine abnormalities, maternal endocrine causes, immunologic causes,

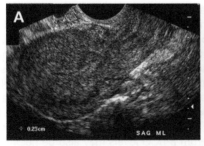
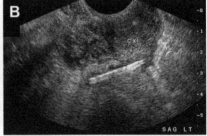

Fig. 16. Perforation of the myometrial wall by an IUD with extrusion into the peritoneal cavity. This 31-year-old woman presented with pelvic pain 5 years status–post insertion of an IUD. (*A*) Midline sagittal EVUS of the uterus reveals no evidence of an IUD within the endometrial cavity (*calipers*). (*B*) Sagittal EVUS reveals the linear echogenic IUD posterior to the cervix (cx) in the cul-de-sac surrounded by a small amount of complex fluid. It has been completely extruded through the myometrial wall.

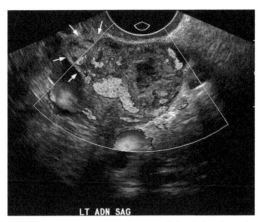

Fig. 17. Corpus luteum. Color Doppler EVUS image of the left adnexal reveals an exophytic CL arising from the left ovary (*arrows*). The wall is thick, homogenous, hypoechoic, and vascular. As the CL involutes, the central cystic component may develop a star-like configuration with internal echoes due to debris and hemorrhage.

and infectious causes.[35] The most common presenting symptoms are pelvic pain, cramping, or vaginal bleeding. The sonographic findings depend on the gestational age. In symptomatic pregnant patients, US examination has an important role in differentiating SAB or fetal demise from a viable IUP or EP. In patients with a suspected SAB, EVUS can be useful in determining whether or not macroscopic tissue remains, which may influence patient management. The presence of an abnormal distorted gestational sac or tissue demonstrating trophoblastic flow, characterized by increased diastolic and systolic velocity, suggests an incomplete abortion **(Fig. 19)**.[36] The EVUS criterion for embryonic demise is the absence of cardiac activity as documented by 2 or more observers for 1 to 3 minutes in an embryo with a crown-rump length

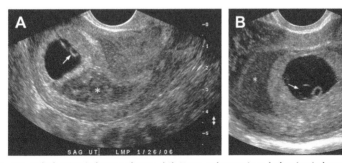

Fig. 18. Subchorionic hemorrhage. (*A*) Note echogenic subchorionic hemorrhage (*asterisk*) in this asymptomatic patient. The subchorionic hemorrhage is adjacent to and slightly larger than the intrauterine gestational sac, which contains a yolk sac (*arrow*). Approximately 25% of the perimeter of the gestational sac is undermined by the subchorionic hemorrhage in this imaging plane. (*B*) This second patient presented with vaginal bleeding in the first trimester. The subchorionic hemorrhage (*asterisk*) is hypoechoic and, although smaller in volume than the gestational sac (*calipers*), undermines close to 75% of the perimeter. Note empty amnion (*arrow*) without evidence of an embryo, another poor prognostic sign, next to the yolk sac.

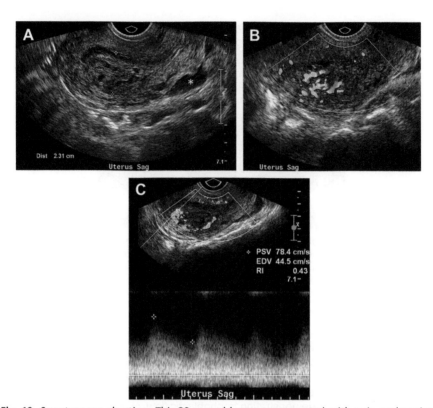

Fig. 19. Spontaneous abortion. This 29-year-old woman presented with pain and vaginal bleeding in the first trimester. (*A*) Sagittal EVUS images of the uterus. Note thickened (2.3-cm) heterogenous endometrial stripe (*calipers*) and a small amount of free fluid in the cul-de-sac (*asterisk*). Findings are nonspecific on gray-scale imaging and could represent hemorrhage or retained products. Color Doppler image (*B*) and spectral tracing (*C*) demonstrate a large amount of vascularity with a low-resistance arterial waveform pattern within the heterogeneous material distending the endometrial canal consistent with retained trophoblastic tissue.

greater than 5 to 6 mm. A complete abortion is defined as complete expulsion of products. In this case, the endometrial cavity is empty or may contain hemorrhage or debris, but no products of conception or trophoblastic flow are seen.[35,36]

Ectopic Pregnancy

EP results when a fertilized oocyte implants outside the endometrial cavity. Although EPs are most commonly located in the ampullary segment of the fallopian tube, ectopic implantation can occur, in order of decreasing frequency, in the isthmic, fimbrial, or interstitial portions of the fallopian tube, ovary, cervix, myometrial scars, and peritoneal cavity (intra-abdominal EP).[37] The possibility of EP should be considered in any woman of reproductive age who presents with acute pelvic pain and a positive β-hCG level. The most recent reports indicate that EPs account for approximately 2% of all pregnancies.[38] Although the mortality rate from EPs has declined in recent years, it remains the most common cause, accounting for 9%, of pregnancy-related deaths in the first trimester.[39] Risk factors for EP include history of prior EP, PID, infertility treatment, prior pelvic surgery, endometriosis, and pregnancy that occurs after placement of an IUD.[40] Although patients with EPs can be asymptomatic, EPs more commonly present with pelvic pain, vaginal bleeding, a palpable adnexal mass, or peritoneal signs. Evaluation for suspected EP should begin with a quantitative measurement of serum β-hCG levels and EVUS.[41,42]

The first step in an EVUS examination performed to evaluate for EP should be to assess for an IUP because most (>70%) symptomatic pregnant patients are found to have an IUP. In patients without significant risk factors for EP, the risk of a coexisting IUP and EP (ie, heterotopic pregnancies) is rare, estimated at between 1/7000 and 1/30,000 pregnancies.[9,43,44] An IUP should be seen on EVUS by 5 weeks gestational age or once the β-hCG level reaches 1000 to 2000 mIU/mL.[41] An eccentric location, within the anterior or posterior layer of the endometrium, of a round anechoic structure with an echogenic rim describes the initial appearance of an IUP on US examination and is termed, *the intradecidual sign*.[45] Once the mean sac diameter of an IUP is greater than or equal to 10 mm, the double decidual sac sign should be present.[46] This refers to the presence of 2 echogenic rings surrounding part of the anechoic gestational sac. The 2 echogenic rings represent the decidua capsularis and decidua parietalis. The hypoechoic area in-between the 2 layers represents a small amount of hypoechoic fluid in the endometrial cavity. If no IUP is seen in a pregnant woman, the diagnostic possibilities include an early IUP of less than 5 weeks' gestational age, embryonic demise or miscarriage, and EP. If the serum β-hCG level is greater than 2000 mIU/mL and no IUP is seen, an EP must be strongly considered even in the absence of adnexal findings, although the diagnostic possibilities include SAB or multiple IUPs.[9,47–50]

The most specific sonographic finding of an EP is the presence of an extrauterine gestational sac containing a yolk sac or embryo (**Fig. 20**).[49–51] An empty tubal ring is the next most specific finding. The wall of an EP is typically echogenic and vascular and EPs are most commonly found in the adnexa between the uterus and ovary. The next most common location is in the cul-de-sac. In the absence of an IUP and with a serum β-hCG level greater than 2000 mIU/mL, however, any extraovarian adnexal mass (except a simple cyst) raises suspicion for an EP.[48–51] A pseudogestational sac, caused by decidualized endometrium and fluid within the endometrial cavity, may be found in 10% to 20% of patients.[49,50,52] A pseudogestational sac is distinguished from an early IUP by the central location of the fluid between the anterior

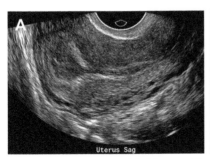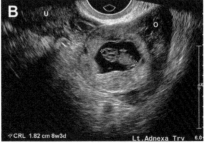

Fig. 20. Ectopic pregnancy. This 24-year-old woman presented with left-sided pelvic pain in the first trimester. (*A*) Sagittal EVUS image of the uterus reveals no evidence of an IUP. (*B*) Image of the left adnexa reveals an extrauterine gestational sac with an echogenic rim containing an embryo (*calipers*). The EP is located between the uterus (U) and left ovary (O). M-mode Doppler revealed a heart rate of 124 beats per minute (not shown).

and posterior endometrial layers and by its elliptical shape.[52] Free fluid may be the only initial sonographic finding in 15% of cases.[51,53] One series reported that 63% of patients with EP had free fluid in the cul-de-sac. Low-level echoes within the free fluid correlates with hemoperitoneum and has been reported in 56% of patients with EP.[54]

It is often difficult to distinguish the empty tubal ring of an EP from an exophytic CL cyst. Both may have an echogenic, vascular wall (ring of fire) and a low-resistance arterial waveform.[31,53,55] Establishing an intraovarian location strongly favors the diagnosis of a CL cyst because intraovarian ectopic pregnancies are rare. Intraovarian location can be confirmed by synchronous movement of the structure with the ovary after manual compression of the ovary during the endovaginal examination or by the demonstration of a small rim of ovarian tissue surrounding the lesion (claw sign).[9] In addition, the wall of the CL tends to be thicker and more homogeneous and hypoechoic than the rim of an EP, although there is overlap in the US appearance.[55,56]

Ovarian Hyperstimulation Syndrome

OHSS is an iatrogenic condition that arises in women undergoing ovulation induction, and occurs during early pregnancy or during the luteal phase of the ovulatory cycle. The incidence of severe OHSS ranges from 0.5% to 5%.[57] In mild cases, both ovaries become enlarged and patients experience mild pelvic discomfort. Abdominal distention, nausea, and vomiting also may occur.[58] In advanced cases, multiple follicles develop and enlarge both ovaries accompanied by third spacing of fluid, especially ascites and pleural effusions. Patients may develop oliguria, tachypnea, and hypotension.[59] The ovaries can grow to more than 10 cm in diameter predisposing them to torsion. Acute pelvic pain in these patients can result from rapid enlargement of a follicle, stretching of the ovarian capsule, hemorrhage into or rupture of a follicle, or ovarian torsion. In 1 series, 60% of pregnant patients who developed ovarian torsion had undergone ovulation induction and had some degree of OHSS.[27] As the ovarian parenchyma is almost completely replaced by many enlarged follicles, the diagnosis of ovarian torsion is difficult in these patients. Sonographic findings in patients with OHSS include markedly enlarged multicystic ovaries (**Fig. 21**A). Debris, retractile clot, or fluid-fluid levels within a cyst suggest hemorrhage (see **Fig. 21**B). Fluid surrounding an ovary or change in shape of a cyst can suggest recent cyst rupture or leakage. Doppler interrogation should always be performed in symptomatic

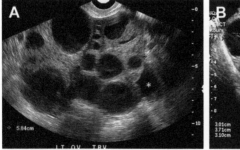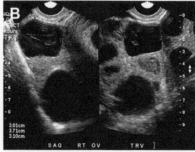

Fig. 21. Ovarian hyperstimulation syndrome. This 37-year-old woman presented with pelvic pain and fullness after ovulation induction. (*A*) Transverse EVUS reveals that both ovaries are massively enlarged (*calipers* = left ovary) and contain many anechoic cysts or follicles. A small amount of free fluid (*asterisk*) is noted adjacent to the left ovary. (*B*) Two weeks later the patient experienced sudden onset of severe pain on the right. Note debris consistent with hemorrhage in one of the right ovarian follicles (*calipers*).

patients to help assess for torsion, although the presence of blood flow does not exclude the diagnosis. Asymmetric size and tenderness should be viewed with suspicion and follow-up MRI may be helpful in confirming the diagnosis of ovarian torsion in these patients. Pelvic ascites can be seen on EVUS, but transabdominal imaging should be performed to evaluate the extent of peritoneal fluid and to look for pleural effusions.

Leiomyomas

Uterine leiomyomas are benign smooth muscle neoplasms reported to occur in up to 40% of women over 30 years old.[60,61] They are commonly associated with dysmennorhea, menorrhagia, chronic pelvic pain and pressure, and infertility. Chronic pelvic pain is usually due to mass effect from large leiomyomas and compression of adjacent structures. Compression of the ureters by an enlarged fibroid uterus, for example, may cause hydronephrosis and flank pain. Leiomyomas are hormonally responsive, and acute pelvic pain can occur when a leiomyoma infarcts or undergoes degeneration, usually after a rapid change in size growing during pregnancy or involuting post partum. Most commonly, a leiomyoma appears as a well-defined hypoechoic mass arising from the myometrium, but the sonographic appearance is variable and leiomyomas can appear echogenic or heterogeneous on US examination. Leiomyomas often demonstrate posterior acoustic shadowing and edge refraction.[62–64] Leiomyomas that have undergone hemorrhagic degeneration during pregnancy tend to demonstrate anechoic cystic spaces and echogenic areas (**Fig. 22**).[65] Pedunculated subserosal leiomyomas can also undergo torsion and become necrotic, which can also be a source of pelvic pain.

PELVIC PAIN IN THE POSTPARTUM PERIOD
Retained Products of Conception

RPOCs complicate approximately 1% of all deliveries but are more common after termination of pregnancy or miscarriage. Patients usually present with vaginal

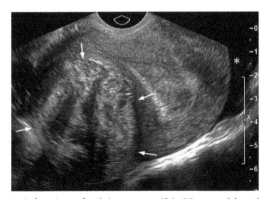

Fig. 22. Hemorrhagic infarction of a leiomyoma. This 28-year-old patient presented with acute, right-sided, pelvic pain in the first trimester. Sagittal EVUS reveals a retroverted uterus, empty endometrial canal, and a moderate amount of free fluid (*asterisk*) near the fundus of the uterus. Note heterogeneous mass (*arrows*) in the anterior wall of the uterus in the region of the patient's pain with areas of increased echogenicity and shadowing. A shadowing myometrial mass most likely represents a leiomyoma. Although leiomyomas may be echogenic on US, in the setting of acute pain this likely represents hemorrhagic infarction. Under the hormonal stimulation of pregnancy, this leiomyoma likely grew rapidly, outstripping its blood supply and infarcting causing sudden-onset, severe, pelvic pain.

bleeding and pelvic pain or cramping.[66] Without treatment, not only do symptoms persist but also pelvic infection and sepsis may develop. Sonographically, RPOCs have a variable appearance, ranging from a heterogenous thick endometrial stripe with trophoblastic flow similar to the US appearance of a patient undergoing miscarriage with residual trophoblastic tissue (see **Fig. 19**) to the presence of an echogenic crescentic mass of placental tissue or fetal parts. The findings are not specific, however, and similar findings can be observed in the normal postpartum uterus.[67,68] Although the diagnosis is made clinically by plateauing of the serum β-hCG level, the finding of visible macroscopic tissue on EVUS can help direct patient management and is suggestive that surgical or pharmacologic completion may be preferable to observation.

Endometritis

Endometritis is a common cause of postpartum pelvic pain and fever and is usually accompanied by leukocytosis and vaginal discharge. Endometritis occurs after cesarean section more commonly than vaginal delivery. Risk factors include prolonged labor, premature rupture of membranes, and RPOCs. The sonographic appearance of endometritis is variable and nonspecific with overlap in the appearance of the normal postpartum endometrium and RPOCs. The endometrium can appear normal or thickened with increased vascularity. Fluid and echogenic debris consistent with hemorrhage or clot are common findings. Echogenic foci with distal shadowing or ring-down artifact may be seen in patients with air in the endometrial cavity, which is concerning for infection (see **Fig. 6**).[66] However, air can normally be seen in the endometrial cavity for up to 3 weeks post delivery up to 3 weeks post delivery, particularly after cesarean section.[69] Hence, clinical correlation with the presence of fever and purulent vaginal discharge is important.

Unusual Causes of Postpartum Pelvic Pain

There are several other, less common, causes of acute pelvic pain in the postpartum period. Ovarian vein thrombophlebitis occurs in less than 2% of patients in the immediate postpartum period. It is more common on the right and after cesarean section. Patients usually present with fever and pain. Sonographic findings may include a tubular or serpiginous avascular mass in the region of the right adnexa and inferior vena cava, lack of color Doppler flow in the right ovarian vein (**Fig. 23**), and thrombus extending to the inferior vena cava, typically better seen with transabdominal imaging. The ovary may be enlarged.[70] Bladder flap hematomas occur in patients after cesarean section and usually appear as a solid complex mass between the posterior bladder wall and anterior wall of the lower uterine segment. These are best seen with transabdominal imaging.[71] Hematomas can also occur in the rectus sheath after cesarean section and are best seen with transabdominal technique using a linear array high-frequency transducer (**Fig. 24**).[72] Finally, uterine rupture is an unusual complication of vaginal delivery, most commonly observed in women who have had prior cesarean section. US usually fails to identify the uterine defect, but can demonstrate intra- or extraperitoneal hematoma and intrauterine hemorrhage (**Fig. 25**).[73]

CHRONIC PELVIC PAIN
Adenomyosis

Adenomyosis is defined as the ectopic location of endometrial glands within the uterine myometrium, usually the inner one-third, with surrounding smooth muscle hyperplasia. Patients present with dysfunctional uterine bleeding, dysmenorrhea,

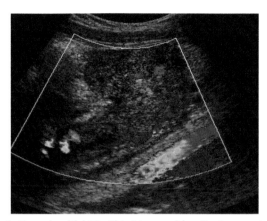

Fig. 23. Ovarian vein thrombophlebitis. This 34-year-old patient presented with abdominal pain and fever 2 days status–post cesarean section. Color Doppler image demonstrates a large tubular structure anterior to the iliac artery (*red*) and vein (*blue*) consistent with a massively dilated gonadal vein almost completely filled with thrombus. Minimal peripheral vascularity is noted.

infertility, or pelvic pain. Adenomyosis is a difficult diagnosis to make clinically because the signs and symptoms are nonspecific and often mimic endometriosis or leiomyomas. The reported frequency of adenomyosis in hysterectomy specimens varies, but the largest series reports an incidence of approximately 20%.[74–76] Adenomyosis occurs more frequently in multiparous women and there is evidence to suggest that it is associated with SAB and dilatation and curettage.[77]

The reported accuracy of EVUS in the detection of adenomyosis varies greatly with sensitivities ranging from 80% to 85% and specificities ranging from 50% to 96%.[78–80] The sonographic appearance of diffuse adenomyosis includes enlargement of the uterus, heterogeneity of the myometrium with poorly marginated heterogeneous hypoechoic or echogenic areas, thickening (especially asymmetric thickening) of the subendometrial halo, asymmetry of the thickness of the anterior and posterior myometrial walls, subendometrial myometrial cysts, echogenic nodules or linear striations extending from the endometrium into the myometrium, and poor definition of the endometrial-myometrial junction (**Fig. 26**). Most studies describe myometrial cysts, which are most commonly visualized in the second half of the menstrual cycle, as the most specific finding on US for adenomyosis.[80–83] These likely represent the

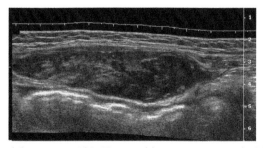

Fig. 24. Rectus sheath hematoma. This 29-year-old woman presented with pain in the anterior abdominal wall 3 days after a cesarean section. Extended field of view US demonstrates a heterogeneous, elliptical hematoma in the rectus muscle.

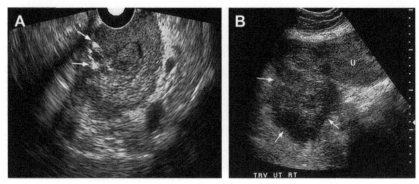

Fig. 25. Uterine rupture. This 25-year-old woman developed excruciating pain 12 hours after the vaginal delivery of her second child. Her first child had been delivered by cesarean section. (*A*) Transverse US image of the lower uterine segment reveals punctate echogenic foci with distal shadowing (*arrows*) in the myometrial wall on the right and debris/hemorrhage within the endometrial cavity. These findings suggest the presence of air and hemorrhage in the cesarean section scar. (*B*) Higher oblique image reveals hemorrhage (*arrows*) dissecting into the broad ligament on the right of the uterus (U). This patient had ruptured her uterus at the site of the cesarean scar.

dilated or hemorrhagic endometrial glands. Another study reported that subendometrial echogenic nodules/radiating striations, representing the ectopic endometrial tissue (see **Fig. 26**), and asymmetric myometrial thickness had the highest positive predictive value in the sonographic diagnosis of adenomyosis.[82,83] Focal adenomyosis or adenomyomas are a less common form of adenomyosis and on US are described as poorly defined myometrial masses with internal vascularity. Rarely, adenomyomas may be cystic. Adenomyosis usually does not alter the outer contour of the uterus.[84,85] Intramural leiomyomas, alternatively, are typically avascular and hypoechoic with well-defined margins. Peripheral vascularity may be noted, especially if the leiomyoma is large.[86] In cases where US is equivocal, MRI increases the diagnostic accuracy.[87,88] Transient myometrial contractions, however, may mimic on US and MRI examination some of these findings, especially thickening of the

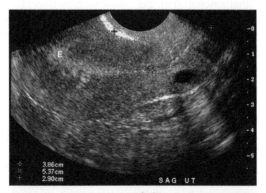

Fig. 26. Adenomyosis. Sagittal EVUS image of the uterus in a 48-year-old woman with menorrhagia reveals nodular and linear echogenic areas extending from the endometrium (E) into the subjacent myometrium consistent with adenomyosis. There is a nabothian cyst in the cervix. Calipers indicate craniocaudad and anteroposterior measurement of the uterus.

subendometrial halo/junctional zone, ill-defined focal hypoechoic areas within the myometrium, and asymmetry in the thickness of the anterior and posterior walls of the uterus.

Endometriosis

Endometriosis is defined as the presence of ectopic endometrial tissue outside of the uterus, most commonly implanted on the surface of the ovary, uterine suspensory ligaments, uterus, or fallopian tube and on the peritoneal surfaces of the pouch of Douglas. Less common sites include the vagina, bladder, cervix, cesarean section scars, abdominal scars, or the inguinal ligament.[86] Under hormonal stimulation, the ectopic endometrium undergoes repeated cycles of hemorrhage, resorption, and fibrosis, resulting in the formation of endometriomas, scarring, and adhesions. Endometriosis has a reported prevalence of 10% in women of reproductive age and has been found in approximately 20% of women undergoing laparoscopy for chronic pelvic pain.[89,90] Risk factors for the development of endometriosis include short menstrual cycles, longer menstrual flow, intermenstrual spotting, and hormone replacement therapy. One half to 80% of patients are symptomatic. Symptoms include dysmenorrhea, dysfunctional uterine bleeding, dyspareunia, infertility, and chronic pelvic pain.[91] Endometriosis is hormonally responsive and pain can be cyclic, related to the menstrual cycle. The degree of pain is not related to the macroscopic extent of disease.

The role of US is limited in the diagnosis of endometriosis because small implants and adhesions are difficult to visualize on US examination. The reported sensitivity of US for the detection of small implants is as low as 11%.[92] Although pelvic MRI is more sensitive than US in the detection of small implants and adhesions, laparoscopy remains the gold standard for diagnosis and staging.[93]

EVUS, however, plays an important role in the diagnosis of endometriomas. On US examination, an endometrioma classically appears as a unilocular homogeneously hypoechoic cystic structure with diffuse low-level echoes and increased through transmission (**Fig. 27**).[94] Echogenic mural foci and shading within a cystic ovarian mass are highly suggestive of endometrioma (see **Fig. 27**).[94] Mural or septal nodularity is worrisome for malignancy because clot occurs less commonly in an endometrioma than in a hemorrhagic cyst. Therefore, further evaluation with MRI or surgery should be considered. Rarely, endometriomas can cause severe pain due to rupture (**Fig. 28**). As endometriomas may be fixed within the pelvis by adhesions, they are at risk for rupture after direct trauma.

Pelvic Congestion Syndrome

Pelvic congestion syndrome is reported to cause chronic pelvic pain, which worsens on standing. Retrograde flow through tortuous and dilated pelvic veins that develop secondary to incompetent valves in the ovarian vein is considered the most likely cause.[86,95–97] It is estimated that up to 60% of patients with pelvic varices have symptoms related to the varicosities.[1] EVUS demonstrates multiple dilated veins surrounding the pelvic organs.[97] Direct connection to the arcuate veins in the myometrium, low velocity flow, and increase in diameter after the Valsalva maneuver all are associated with symptoms (**Fig. 29**).[96] The treatment of pelvic congestion syndrome remains controversial, but bilateral transcatheter embolization with sclerotherapy is reported to successfully improve symptoms in some cases, although the durability of the symptomatic improvement is highly variable.

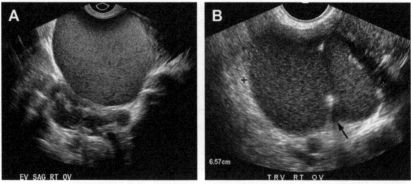

Fig. 27. Endometrioma. This 42-year-old woman presented with chronic pelvic pain. (*A*) Large right adnexal mass with homogeneous low-level echogenicity, the most classic US appearance of an endometrioma. Hypoechoic band anteriorly that gradually becomes more echogenic inferiorly has been described as shading, which is most likely due to gradual settling of blood products and RBCs in the thick viscous fluid within the endometrioma. (*B*) Another patient with endometriosis demonstrates 2 adjacent endometriomas (*calipers*) in the right adnexa. Note angular margins (*arrow*) likely due to scarring or adhesions. Small echogenic linear mural foci are a specific US feature of endometriomas, although the histologic/pathologic correlate is not known.

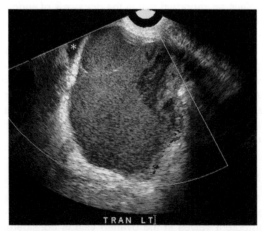

Fig. 28. Rupture of an endometrioma. This patient with known endometriosis presented with sudden onset of severe abdominal pain after a car accident. Endometriomas may be fixed in the pelvis due to scarring and adhesions and large endometriomas therefore may be at risk to rupture after direct trauma. EVUS color Doppler image of the left adnexal demonstrates a mass that is largely homogenous with low-level echoes consistent with the diagnosis of an endometrioma. Note, however, the irregular contour and adjacent free fluid (*asterisk*). More echogenic free fluid, consistent with hemoperitoneum was noted in the cul-de-sac (not shown). At surgery the endometrioma had ruptured, leaking its contents into the peritoneal cavity.

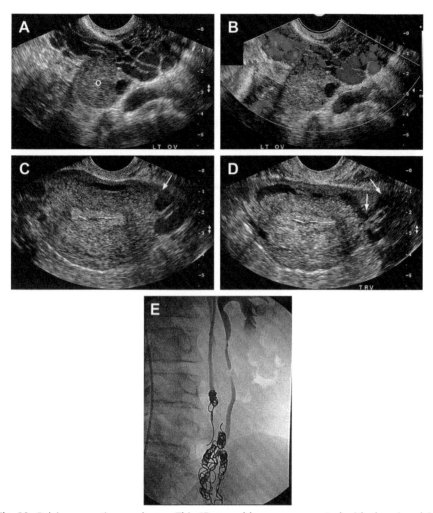

Fig. 29. Pelvic congestion syndrome. This 45-year-old woman presented with chronic pelvic pain. Gray-scale (*A*) and color Doppler image (*B*) reveal many dilated veins in the left adnexa. Left ovary (O). (*C, D*) The enlarged pelvic veins directly communicated with the arcuate veins (*arrows*) within the myometrium. Pelvic venogram demonstrated reflux in the gonadal vein consistent with pelvic congestion syndrome. The patient underwent coil embolization and sclerotherapy of the pelvic varices and gonadal veins (coils in the *left* gonadal veins shown in [*E*]) with relief of her symptoms.

SUMMARY

US should be considered the first-line imaging modality of choice in women presenting with acute or chronic pelvic pain of suspected gynecologic or obstetric origin because many, if not most, gynecologic/obstetric causes of pelvic pain are easily diagnosed on US examination. Since the clinical presentation of gynecologic causes of pelvic pain overlaps with gastrointestinal and genitourinary pathology, however, referral to CT or MRI, especially in pregnant patients, should be considered if the US examination is nondiagnostic.

ACKNOWLEDGMENTS

The authors would like to thank Ms Geri Mancini for her expert help with image preparation.

REFERENCES

1. Andreotti RF, Lee SI, Choy G, et al. ACR Appropriateness Criteria on acute pelvic pain in the reproductive age group. J Am Coll Radiol 2009;6:235–41.
2. Mathias SD, Kuppermann M, Liberman RF, et al. Chronic pelvic pain: prevalence, health-related quality of life, and economic correlates. Obstet Gynecol 1996; 87(3):321–7.
3. Howard FM. The role of laparoscopy in chronic pelvic pain: promise and pitfall. Obstet Gynecol Surv 1993;48:357–87.
4. Sharma D, Dahiya K, Duhan N, et al. Diagnostic laparoscopy in chronic pelvic pain. Arch Gynaecol Obstet Jan 2010. [online].
5. Burnett LS. Gynecologic causes of the acute abdomen. Surg Clin North Am 1988; 68:385–516.
6. Borgfeldt C, Andolf E. Transvaginal sonographic ovarian findings in a random sample of women 25–40 years old. Ultrasound Obstet Gynecol 1999;13:345–50.
7. Ekerhovd E, Wienerroith H, Staudach A, et al. Preoperative assessment of uniloc-ular adnexal cysts by transvaginal ultrasonography: a comparison between ultra-sonographic morphologic imaging and histopathologic diagnosis. Am J Obstet Gynecol 2001;184(2):48–54.
8. Levine D, Brown D. Report from the SRU Consensus Conference on Management of asymptomatic ovarian and other adnexal cysts imaged on ultrasound. Radi-ology, in press.
9. Scoutt LM. Sonographic evaluation of acute pelvic pain in women. In State-of- the-art emergency and trauma radiology: ARRS categorical course syllabus; 2008. p. 229–40.
10. Hertzberg BS, Kliewer MA, Paulson EK. Ovarian cyst rupture causing hemoper-itoneum: imaging features and the potential for misdiagnosis. Abdom Imaging 1999;24:304–8.
11. Hertzberg BS, Kliewer MA, Bowie JD. Adnexal ring sign and hemoperitoneum caused by hemorrhagic ovarian cyst: pitfall in the sonographic diagnosis of ectopic pregnancy. Am J Roentgenol 1999;173:1301–2.
12. Jain KA. Sonographic spectrum of hemorrhagic ovarian cysts. J Ultrasound Med 2002;21:879–86.
13. Barret S, Taylor C. A review on pelvic inflammatory disease. Int J STD AIDS 2005; 16:715–21.
14. Patten RM, Vincent LM, Wolner-Hanssen P, et al. Pelvic inflammatory disease. Endovaginal sonography with laparoscopic correlation. J Ultrasound Med 1990;9:681–9.
15. Timor-Tristsch IE, Lerner JP, Mongeagudo A, et al. Transvaginal sonographic markers of tubal inflammatory disease. Ultrasound Obstet Gynecol 1998;12: 56–66.
16. Horrow M. Ultrasound of pelvic inflammatory disease. Ultrasound Q 2004;20: 171–9.
17. Hibbard LT. Adnexal torsion. Am J Obstet Gynecol 1985;152:456–61.
18. Albayram F, Hamper UM. Ovarian and adnexal torsion: spectrum of sonographic findings with pathologic correlation. J Ultrasound Med 2001;20:1063–9.

19. Chen M, Chen C, Yang Y. Torsion of the previously normal uterine adnexa. Evaluation of the correlation between the pathologic changes and the clinical characteristics. Acta Obstet Gynecol Scand 2001;80:58–61.
20. Argenta PA, Yeagley TJ, Ott G, et al. Torsion of the uterine adnexa. Pathologic correlations and current management trends. J Reprod Med 2000;45:831–6.
21. Houry D, Abbott JT. Ovarian torsion: a fifteen-year review. Ann Emerg Med 2001; 38:156–9.
22. White M, Stella J. Ovarian torsion: 10-year perspective. Emerg Med Australas 2005;17:231–7.
23. Graif M, Shalev J, Strauss J, et al. Torsion of the ovary: sonographic features. Am J Roentgenol 1984;143:1331–4.
24. Lee EJ, Kwon HC, Joo HJ, et al. Diagnosis of ovarian torsion with color Doppler sonography: depiction of twisted vascular pedicle. J Ultrasound Med 1998;17: 83–9.
25. Vijayaraghavan SB. Sonographic whirlpool sign in ovarian torsion. J Ultrasound Med 2004;23:1643–9.
26. Ben-Ami M, Perlitz Y, Haddad S. The effectiveness of spectral and color Doppler in predicting ovarian torsion. A prospective study. Eur J Obstet Gynecol Reprod Biol 2002;104:64–6.
27. Pena J, Ufberg D, Cooney N, et al. Usefulness of Doppler sonography in the diagnosis of ovarian torsion. Fertil Steril 2000;73:1047–50.
28. Fleischer AC, Stein SM, Cullinan JA, et al. Color Doppler sonography of adnexal torsion. J Ultrasound Med 1995;14:523–8.
29. Pellerito JS, Troiano RN, Quedens-Case C, et al. Common pitfalls of endovaginal color Doppler flow imaging. Radiographics 1995;15:37–47.
30. Benacerraf BR, Shipp TD, Bromley B. Three-dimensional ultrasound detection of abnormally located intrauterine contraceptive devices which are a source of pelvic pain and abnormal bleeding. Ultrasound Obstet Gynecol 2009;34:110–5.
31. Durfee SM, Frates MC. Sonographic spectrum of the corpus luteum in early pregnancy: gray-scale, color, and pulsed Doppler appearance. J Clin Ultrasound 1999;27:55–9.
32. Abu-Yousef MM, Bleicher JJ, Williamson RA, et al. Subchorionic hemorrhage: sonographic diagnosis and clinical significance. Am J Roentgenol 1987;149:737–40.
33. Bennett GL, Bromley B, Lieberman E, et al. Subchorionic hemorrhage in first-trimester pregnancies: prediction of pregnancy outcome with sonography. Radiology 1996;200:803–6.
34. Sauerbrei EE, Pham DH. Placental abruption and subchorionic hemorrhage in the first half of pregnancy: US appearance and clinical outcome. Radiology 1986; 160:109–12.
35. Dighe M, Cuevas C, Moshiri M, et al. Sonography in first trimester bleeding. J Clin Ultrasound 2008;36:352–66.
36. Nyberg DA, Laing FC, Filly RA. Threatened abortion: sonographic distinction of normal and abnormal gestation sacs. Radiology 1986;158:397–400.
37. Bouyer J, Coste J, Fernandez H, et al. Sites of ectopic pregnancy: a 10 year population-based study of 1800 cases. Hum Reprod 2002;17:3224–30.
38. Centers for disease control and prevention. Ectopic pregnancy—United States, 1990–1992. MMWR Morb Mortal Wkly Rep 1995;44:46–8.
39. Chang J, Elam-Evans JD, Berg CJ, et al. Pregnancy related mortality surveillance—United States, 1991–1999. MMWR Surveill Summ 2003;52:1–9.
40. Barnhart KT, Sammel MD, Gracia CR, et al. Risk factors for ectopic pregnancy in women with symptomatic first-trimester pregnancies. Fertil Steril 2006;86:36–43.

41. Carson SA, Buster JE. Ectopic pregnancy. N Engl J Med 1993;329:1174–81.
42. Barnhart KT. Ectopic pregnancy. N Engl J Med 2009;361:379–87.
43. Hann LE, Bachman DM, McArdle CR. Coexistent intrauterine and ectopic pregnancy: a reevaluation. Radiology 1984;152:151–4.
44. Anastasakis E, Jetti A, Macara L, et al. A case of heterotopic pregnancy in the absence of risk factors. A brief literature review. Fetal Diagn Ther 2007;22:285–8.
45. Yeh HC, Goodman JL, Carr L, et al. Intradecidual sign: is it effective in diagnosis of an early intrauterine pregnancy? Radiology 1997;204:655–60.
46. Bradley WG, Friske CE, Filly RA. The double decidual sac sign of early intrauterine pregnancy: use in exclusion of ectopic pregnancy. Radiology 1982;143: 223–6.
47. Cacciatore B, Stenman UH, Ylostalo P. Diagnosis of ectopic pregnancy by vaginal ultrasonography in combination with discriminatory serum beta-hCG level of 1000 IU/l IRP. Br J Obstet Gynaecol 1990;97:904–8.
48. Atri M, Leduc C, Gillett P, et al. Role of endovaginal sonography in the diagnosis and management of ectopic pregnancy. Radiographics 1996;16:755–74.
49. Lin EP, Bhatt S, Dogra VS. Diagnostic clues to ectopic pregnancy. Radiographics 2008;28:1661–71.
50. Levine D. Ectopic pregnancy. Radiology 2007;245:385–97.
51. Brown DL, Doubilet PM. Transvaginal sonography for diagnosing ectopic pregnancy: positivity criteria and performance characteristics. J Ultrasound Med 1994;13:259–66.
52. Dillon EF, Feyock AL, Taylor KJ. Pseudogestational sacs: Doppler differentiation from normal or abnormal intrauterine pregnancies. Radiology 1990;176:359–64.
53. Pellerito JS, Taylor KJ, Quedens-Case C, et al. Ectopic pregnancy: evaluation with endovaginal color flow imaging. Radiology 1992;183:407–11.
54. Nyberg DA, Hughes MP, Mack LA, et al. Extrauterine findings of ectopic pregnancy at transvaginal US: importance of echogenic fluid. Radiology 1991;178: 823–6.
55. Frates MC, Visweswaran A, Laing FC. Comparison of tubal ring and corpus luteum echogenicities; useful differentiating characteristics. J Ultrasound Med 2001;20:27–31.
56. Stein MW, Ricci ZJ, Novak L, et al. Sonographic comparison of the tubal ring of ectopic pregnancy with the corpus luteum. J Ultrasound Med 2004;23:57–62.
57. Delvigne A, Rozenberg S. Epidemiology and prevention of ovarian hyperstimulation syndrome (OHSS): a review. Hum Reprod Update 2002;8:559–77.
58. Practice Committee of the American Society for Reproductive Medicine. Ovarian hyperstimulation syndrome. Fertil Steril 2008;90:S188–93.
59. Bergh PA, Navot D. Ovarian hyperstimulation syndrome: a review of pathophysiology. J Assist Reprod Genet 1992;9:429–38.
60. Wallach EE, Vlahos NF. Uterine myomas: an overview of development, clinical features, and management. Obstet Gynecol 2004;104:393–406.
61. Stewart EA. Uterine fibroids. Lancet 2001;357:293–8.
62. Sheth S, Macura K. Sonography of the uterine myometrium: myomas and beyond. Ultrasound Clin 2007;2:267–95.
63. Mayer DP, Shipilov V. Ultrasonography and magnetic resonance imaging of uterine fibroids. Obstet Gynecol Clin North Am 1995;22:667–725.
64. Karasick S, Lev-Toaff AS, Toaff ME. Imaging of uterine leiomyomas. Am J Roentgenol 1992;158:799–805.
65. Lev-Toaff AS, Coleman BG, Arger PH, et al. Leiomyomas in pregnancy: sonographic study. Radiology 1987;164:375–80.

66. Zukerman J, Levine D, McNicholas MM, et al. Imaging of pelvic postpartum complications. Am J Roentgenol 1997;168:663–8.
67. Sadan O, Golan A, Girtler O, et al. Role of sonography in the diagnosis of retained products of conception. J Ultrasound Med 2004;23:371–4.
68. Dufree SM, Frates MC, Luong A, et al. The sonographic and color Doppler features of retained products of conception. J Ultrasound Med 2005;24:1181–6.
69. Brown DL. Pelvic ultrasound in the postabortion and postpartum patient. Ultrasound Q 2005;21:27–37.
70. Savader SJ, Otero RR, Savader BL. Puerperal ovarian vein thrombosis: evaluation with CT, US, and MR imaging. Radiology 1988;167:637–9.
71. Baker ME, Bowie JD, Killam AP. Sonography of post-cesarian-section bladder-flap hematoma. Am J Roentgenol 1985;144:757–9.
72. Wiener MD, Bowie JD, Baker ME, et al. Sonography of subfascial hematoma after cesarean delivery. Am J Roentgenol 1987;148:907–10.
73. Has R, Topuz S, Kalelioglu I, et al. Imaging features of postpartum uterine rupture: a case report. Abdom Imaging 2008;33:101–3.
74. Azziz R. Adenomyosis: current perspectives. Obstet Gynecol Clin North Am 1989;16:221–35.
75. Vercellini P, Parazzini F, Oldani S, et al. Adenomyosis at hysterectomy: a study on frequency distribution and patient characteristics. Hum Reprod 1995;10:1160–2.
76. Vercellini P, Vigano P, Somigliana E, et al. Adenomyosis: epidemiological factors. Best Pract Res Clin Obstet Gynaecol 2006;20:465–77.
77. Levgur M, Abadi MA, Tucker A. Adenomyosis: symptoms, histology, and pregnancy terminations. Obstet Gynecol 2000;95:688–91.
78. Bromley B, Shipp TD, Benacerraf B. Adenomyosis: sonographic findings and diagnostic accuracy. J Ultrasound Med 2000;19:529–34.
79. Dueholm M. Transvaginal ultrasound for diagnosis of adenomyosis: a review. Best Pract Res Clin Obstet Gynaecol 2006;20:569–82.
80. Reinhold C, Tafazoli F, Mehio A, et al. Endovaginal US and MR imaging features with histopathologic correlation. Radiographics 1999;19:S147–60.
81. Bazot M, Cortez A, Darai E, et al. Ultrasonography compared with magnetic resonance imaging for the diagnosis of adenomyosis: correlation with histopathology. Hum Reprod 2001;16:2427–33.
82. Atri M, Reinhold C, Mehio A, et al. Adenomyosis: US features with histologic correlation in an in-vitro study. Radiology 2000;215:783–90.
83. Reinhold C, Tafazoli F, Wang L. Imaging features of adenomyosis. Hum Reprod Update 1998;4:337–49.
84. Andreotti RF, Fleischer AC. The sonographic diagnosis of adenomyosis. Ultrasound Q 2005;21:167–70.
85. Bostis D, Kassanos D, Antoniou G, et al. Adenomyoma and leiomyoma: differential diagnosis with transvaginal sonography. J Clin Ultrasound 1998;26:21–5.
86. Kuligowska E, Deeds L, Lu K. Pelvic pain: overlooked and underdiagnosed gynecologic conditions. Radiographics 2005;25:3–20.
87. Ascher SM, Arnold LL, Patt RH, et al. Adenomyosis: prospective comparison of MR imaging and transvaginal sonography. Radiology 1994;190:803–6.
88. Dueholm M, Lundorf E. Transvaginal ultrasond or MRI for diagnosis of adenomyosis. Curr Opin Obstet Gynecol 2007;19:505–12.
89. Mahmood TA, Templeton A. Prevalence and genesis of endometriosis. Hum Reprod 1991;6:544–9.
90. El-Yahia AW. Laparoscopic evaluation of apparently normal infertile women. Aust N Z J Obstet Gynaecol 1994;34:440–2.

91. Rawson JM. Prevalence of endometriosis in asymptomatic women. J Reprod Med 1991;36:513–5.
92. Friedman H, Vogelzang RL, Mendelson EB, et al. Endometriosis detection by US with laparoscopic correlation. Radiology 1985;157:217–20.
93. Dubela AJ. Diagnosis of endometriosis. Obstet Gynecol Clin North Am 1997;24: 331–46.
94. Patel MD, Feldstein VA, Chen DC, et al. Endometriomas: diagnostic performance of US. Radiology 1999;210:739–45.
95. Beard RW, Reginald PW, Wadsworth J. Clinical features of women with chronic lower abdominal pain and pelvic congestion. Br J Obstet Gynaecol 1988;95: 153–61.
96. Park SJ, Lim LW, Ko YT, et al. Diagnosis of pelvic congestion syndrome using transabdominal and transvaginal sonography. Am J Roentgenol 2004;182:683–8.
97. Ganeshan A, Upponi S, Hon LQ, et al. Chronic pelvic pain due to pelvic congestion syndrome: the role of diagnostic and interventional radiology. Cardiovasc Intervent Radiol 2007;30:1105–11.

Ultrasound Assessment of Premenopausal Bleeding

Raj M. Paspulati, MD[a], Ahmet T. Turgut, MD[b,c],
Shweta Bhatt, MD[d], Elif Ergun, MD[b], Vikram S. Dogra, MD[d,*]

KEYWORDS

- Pregnancy • Abortion • Arteriovenous malformation
- Bleeding • Ultrasound • First trimester

First trimester pregnancy accounts for the majority of patients with premenopausal bleeding. In the first trimester of pregnancy, 25% of women experience vaginal bleeding. Nearly 50% of these women have an abnormal outcome, while the other 50% continue to term.[1] The differentiation between these two groups depends upon the identification of a normal intrauterine gestation in this early stage of pregnancy; thus, the radiologist must be familiar with the normal appearance of intrauterine gestation at various stages of first trimester pregnancy. It is important to recognize the sonographic appearance of abnormal intrauterine gestation and intrauterine changes of an ectopic pregnancy. Before the embryonic stage of pregnancy, a combination of serum quantitative beta human chorionic gonadotropin (hCG) and transvaginal ultrasonography (TVUS) is an accurate method of identifying a normal intrauterine gestation. The concept of the discriminatory zone, which is the serum beta hCG level at which an intrauterine gestation should be seen by TVUS, is an important landmark in identifying a normal intrauterine pregnancy.[2,3] This discriminatory zone varies between 1,000 IU/mL to 2,000 IU/mL and is commonly cited to be at 1,500 IU/mL.[2,4] The normal intrauterine gestational sac (GS), before the appearance of the yolk sac (YS), has a double decidual sac appearance because of the separation of the decidua capsularis overlying the GS from the deciduas parietalis by the endometrial cavity.[5,6] Identification of a YS within the GS is a definitive sign of

A version of this article was previously published in *Ultrasound Clinics* 3:3.
[a] Department of Radiology, University Hospitals, Case Medical Center, Case Western Reserve University 11100 Euclid Avenue, Cleveland, OH 44106, USA
[b] Department of Radiology, Ankara Training and Research Hospital, TR-06590, Ankara, Turkey
[c] 25. Cadde, 362. Sokak, Hüner Sitesi No: 18/30, TR-06530, Ankara, Turkey
[d] Department of Imaging Sciences, University of Rochester School of Medicine, 601 Elmwood Avenue, Box 648, Rochester, NY 14642, USA
* Corresponding author.
E-mail address: vikram_dogra@urmc.rochester.edu

Obstet Gynecol Clin N Am 38 (2011) 115–147
doi:10.1016/j.ogc.2011.02.006
0889-8545/11/$ – see front matter © 2011 Elsevier Inc. All rights reserved.

obgyn.theclinics.com

intrauterine gestation.[7,8] An ectopic pregnancy is strongly considered when an extra ovarian adnexal mass is observed without an intrauterine GS and serum beta hCG is above the discriminatory level. Demonstration of an extrauterine GS with a YS or embryo is a definitive sign of an ectopic pregnancy. Hydatidiform mole is a more common manifestation of gestational trophoblastic disease (GTD), which is a spectrum of pregnancy-related proliferative trophoblastic abnormalities. A high or rapidly rising serum beta hCG and a complex intrauterine mass with cystic foci is indicative of a molar pregnancy. Arteriovenous malformation (AVM) is a rare but important cause of first trimester bleeding, and distinguishing this entity from retained products of gestation is vital, as its management is entirely different.[9,10] Important causes of first trimester bleeding are spontaneous abortion, ectopic pregnancy, gestational trophoblastic disease, and AVM.

This article provides an overview of ultrasound (US) scanning techniques, the normal sonographic landmarks of intrauterine gestation, and sonographic features of an abnormal intrauterine gestation in spontaneous abortion, ectopic pregnancy, GTD, and AVM of the uterus, accounting for premenopausal bleeding.

ULTRASOUND SCANNING TECHNIQUES

In women presenting with first trimester bleeding, transabdominal ultrasound (TAUS) with a 3.5-MHz transducer is initially performed with a full bladder to displace the bowel and provide an acoustic window. This provides a general overview of the uterus and adnexa. After the bladder is emptied, TVUS is performed using a 5-MHz to 10-MHz transducer. Higher frequency US and the closer position of the transducer to the imaging structures provides high-resolution images of the uterus and adnexa, which is essential to detect early intrauterine gestation and abnormalities associated with first trimester bleeding. Color flow Doppler and pulsed Doppler US should be used if necessary, but one should keep in mind the concept of "as low as reasonably achievable" to avoid potential harmful effects on the developing embryo.[11]

NORMAL SONOGRAPHIC LANDMARKS OF INTRAUTERINE GESTATION

Normal sonographic milestones of first trimester pregnancy are shown in **Table 1**. Approximately 1 week after fertilization, the blastocyst is implanted in the endometrium and is too small to be visualized by TVUS. Focal thickening of the endometrium with an increased trophoblastic flow on color flow Doppler at the implanted site is reported to be the earliest sign of an intrauterine gestation, but is a nonspecific and unreliable sign.[12] An eccentric anechoic focus within the thickened endometrium, described as an "intradecidual sign," is the earliest evidence of an implanted blastocyst (**Fig. 1**).[13]

Table 1 Normal sonographic milestones of first trimester pregnancy		
Parameter	**Transabdominal US**	**Transvaginal US**
Gestational sac	–	Present at 5 weeks
Yolk sac	Always present with a MSD of >16 mm	Always present with a MSD of >8 mm
Embryo	Always present with a MSD of >25 mm	Always present with a MSD of >16 mm
Embryonic cardiac activity	CRL of >5 mm	CRL of >5 mm

Abbreviations: CRL, crown rump length; GS, gestational sac; MSD, mean sac diameter.

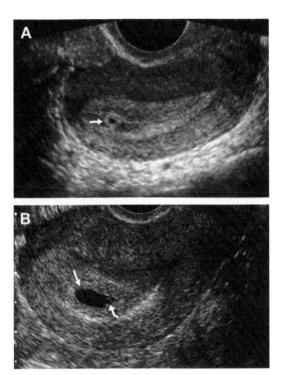

Fig. 1. Intradecidual sign. (*A*) Sagittal TVUS of the uterus demonstrates an eccentric anechoic focus (*arrow*) in the endometrial lining representing early blastocyst. (*B*) Follow up TVUS after two weeks shows a well-defined gestational sac (*arrow*) with a yolk sac (*curved arrow*) confirming an intrauterine gestation.

Gestational Sac

GS is the sonographic term for the fluid-filled chorionic cavity of the implanted blastocyst. It is seen as early as the first 4 weeks of gestational age as a 2-mm to 3-mm eccentric sonolucent focus with a surrounding echogenic rim formed by the combined trophoblastic and decidual reaction. This surrounding rim of a normal GS is more echogenic than the myometrium and is 2-mm to 3-mm thick (**Fig. 2**).[1] The double decidual sac sign (DDS) of a true intrauterine GS is caused by eccentric GS in the endometrium surrounded by the ipsilateral decidua basalis and decidua capsularis, which is separated from the decidua parietalis by the collapsed endometrial cavity (**Fig. 3**). This appearance distinguishes a true intrauterine GS before the appearance of a YS from a pseudogestational sac of ectopic pregnancy, which is caused by fluid in the endometrial cavity surrounded by thick decidual reaction.[5,6]

Yolk Sac

The secondary YS is the first extraembryonic structure to be seen by TVUS within the GS (chorionic cavity). It is visualized at 5 weeks and is the first reliable sign of intrauterine gestation. It is a well-defined, thin walled cystic structure that gradually increases in size from 5 to 11 weeks of gestation and reaches a maximum size of 5 mm to 6 mm; it is generally not seen after 12 weeks. In a normal intrauterine gestation, a YS should be seen when the mean sac diameter (MSD) is 8 mm (**Fig. 4**). The YS

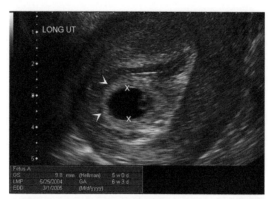

Fig. 2. Sagittal TVUS of the uterus shows a normal gestational sac (*within the calipers*) with a thick echogenic rim representing chorionic villi and decidual reaction (*arrowheads*).

is located between the amnion and chorion and is connected to the embryo by a stalk-like vitelline or omphalomesenteric duct.[7,8,14]

Embryo

The earliest evidence of an embryo is seen as a focal thickening at the periphery of adjoining the YS (see **Fig. 4**). With the currently available high-frequency transducers, embryonic cardiac activity is often appreciated adjacent to the YS, even before an embryo is well visualized.[15–17] An embryo should always be seen by TVUS when the MSD of the GS is 16 mm and by TAUS when the MSD is 25 mm (**Fig. 5**).[7,14] Cardiac activity should always be seen and documented in all embryos with a crown rump length (CRL) of 5 mm.[18,19] Cardiac activity increases gradually from 100 beats per minute (bpm) at 5 to 6 weeks gestation to about 140 bpms at 8 to 9 weeks of gestation and should be documented by M-mode.[20]

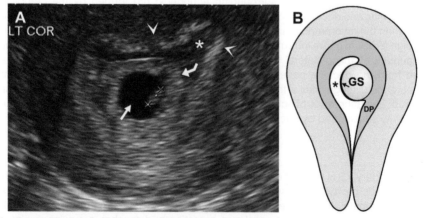

Fig. 3. Double decidual sac sign. (*A*) Coronal TVUS of the uterus reveals an intrauterine gestational sac (*arrow*), decidua capsularis (*curved arrow*), decidua parietalis (*arrowhead*), and effaced endometrial cavity (*asterisk*). (*B*) The corresponding line diagram.

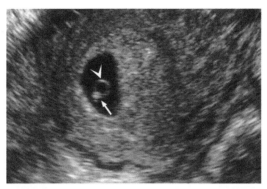

Fig. 4. TVUS of the uterus at 5-weeks menstrual age demonstrates an intrauterine gestational sac with a yolk sac (*arrowhead*) and an echogenic focus (*arrow*) adjacent to the yolk sac representing an early embryo.

Chorio-Amniotic Membranes

The amniotic sac is formed at about 4 weeks of gestation and is visible by TVUS at 5 to 6 weeks as a separate cystic structure, separated from the YS by the embryonic disc. This appearance has been described as "the double bleb sign."[21] The amniotic sac gradually enlarges and completely surrounds the embryo and the YS is located outside the amniotic sac. The amniotic membrane is less than 0.5-mm thick and is best seen when the US beam is perpendicular to the membrane.[21] The amniotic sac gradually increases in size and fuses with the outer chorionic membrane between 14 and 16 weeks of gestation. Before 6.5 weeks of gestation, the amniotic membrane is closely aligned to the embryo and is not readily seen by TVUS. Separation of the amniotic and chorionic membranes is a normal feature before 14 weeks of gestation and is abnormal after 17 weeks.[22,23] The contents of the amniotic sac are anechoic; low-level echoes and linear strands can normally be seen within the chorionic cavity outside the amniotic membrane. This is because of high proteinaceous contents, coagulum, and mesodermal strands (**Fig. 6**).[21]

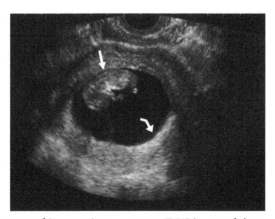

Fig. 5. Embryonic stage of intrauterine pregnancy. TVUS image of the uterus at 7 weeks of menstrual age demonstrates a well-developed embryo (*arrow*) within a gestational sac (*curved arrow*).

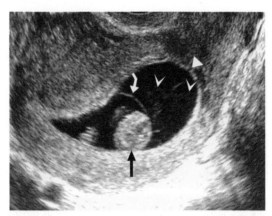

Fig. 6. Sagittal TVUS of the uterus demonstrates intrauterine pregnancy with an embryo (*arrow*), thin amniotic membrane (*curved arrow*) adjacent to the embryo, and a peripheral thick chorionic membrane (*solid arrowhead*). The chorionic and amniotic membranes are not yet fused with low level echoes (*arrowheads*) between the unfused chorion and amnion.

SPONTANEOUS ABORTION

Spontaneous abortion is defined as termination of pregnancy during the first 20 weeks of gestation. It is more common in the first 16 weeks of gestation and the incidence decreases as gestational age increases. Genetic abnormalities are the most common cause of spontaneous abortion; autosomal trisomy is the most frequently identified abnormality.[24] Environmental factors account for the remaining small percentage of spontaneous abortions. The causes of spontaneous abortion are displayed in **Box 1**. Spontaneous abortion is classified clinically as threatened, missed, incomplete, and complete abortion.

Threatened abortion is the most common presentation and occurs in 25% of all pregnancies. After confirmation of the pregnancy by a urine pregnancy test and determination of the serum beta hCG levels, the management of these patients depends upon the viability of the gestation. TVUS is necessary to confirm an intrauterine gestation and to assess the viability and probable outcome.

Sonography in Spontaneous Abortion

Knowledge of the normal sonographic milestones of first trimester pregnancy is essential to identify abnormal sonographic features and probable outcomes in these patients. The sonographic findings depend upon the stage of gestation and have to be correlated with serum beta hCG levels. TVUS features of an abnormal gestation are displayed in **Table 2**.

SONOGRAPHIC FEATURES OF ABNORMAL INTRAUTERINE GESTATION
Pre-Embryonic Stage

Correlation of ultrasonographic findings with serum beta hCG is essential in this early stage of gestation. A GS should be identified in the uterus when serum beta hCG has reached the discriminatory level, which ranges from 1,000 IU to 1,500 IU.[2,3,25] The appearance of the GS, YS, and the choriodecidual reaction determines the probable outcome for these patients.

Box 1
Causes of spontaneous abortion

Genetic causes

Trisomy

Aneuploidy/polyploidy, translocations

Environmental causes

Uterus

    Congenital uterine anomalies

    Leiomyoma

    Intrauterine adhesions or synechiae (Asherman's syndrome)

Endocrine

    Progesterone deficiency (inadequate luteal phase)

    Thyroid disease

    Diabetes mellitus (uncontrolled)

    Luteinizing hormone hypersecretion

Immunologic

    Antiphospholipid syndrome, systemic lupus erythematosus (SLE)

Infections

    Toxoplasma gondii,

    Listeria monocytogens,

    Chlamydia trachomatis,

    Ureaplasma urealyticum,

    Mycoplasma hominis,

    Herpes simplex,

    Treponema pallidum,

    Borrelia burgdorferi,

    Neisseria gonorrhoea

Gestational sac criteria

The GS size, shape, and location are important predictors of pregnancy outcome. A GS with an MSD of 8 mm to 10 mm without a YS, and a GS with an MSD of 16 mm to 20 mm without an embryo, is an indicator of abnormal gestation (**Fig. 7**A).[7,26] This empty GS without a YS or embryo is because of early embryonic demise and resorption of the embryo. An abnormal karyotype, such as autosomal trisomy or triploidy, is the cause for this early pregnancy failure. This anembryonic gestation is also called "blighted ovum" and "empty amnion sign" (see **Fig. 7**A; **Fig. 8**).[27,28] A GS small for the gestational age should be followed by US at 1- to 2-week intervals. A small GS with a growth rate of less than 1 mm per day is an indicator for a poor outcome.[29] A distorted GS, low lying GS, the absence of the double decidual sac sign, and thin (<2 mm) decidual reaction are other minor criteria of an abnormal gestation (**Fig. 7**B).[7,26]

Table 2
TVUS features of abnormal outcome in first trimester bleeding

Ultrasound Findings	Comments
Serum beta hCG above discriminatory level (1,000 mIU/mL) without IUGS	Ectopic gestation has to be excluded
MSD of > 8 mm without a yolk sac	Follow-up with serum beta hCG and TVUS
MSD of >16 mm without an embryo	Anembryonic pregnancy
Embryo with CRL of 5 mm and >	Embryonic demise without cardiac activity
Embryo with bradycardia (<100 bpm)	Poor outcome and needs close TVUS follow-up
Small GS with a <5 mm difference between MSD and CRL	Poor out come with embryonic demise or oligohydramnios
Subchorionic hematoma	Correlation of the size of subchorionic hematoma with pregnancy outcome is not well established and needs TVUS follow-up

Abbreviations: bpm, beats per minute; IUGS, intrauterine gestational sac.

Yolk sac criteria

Identification of a YS within the GS is the most reliable sign of intrauterine gestation in the pre-embryonic stage.[7,8] Absence of a YS in the presence of an embryo is an indicator of poor outcome.[14,30] An abnormally large YS (>6 mm) or small, echogenic, and calcified YSs are associated with embryonic death (**Fig. 9**).[31–33] The YS is associated with nutritive, metabolic, and hemopoetic functions of the early embryo. The abnormal

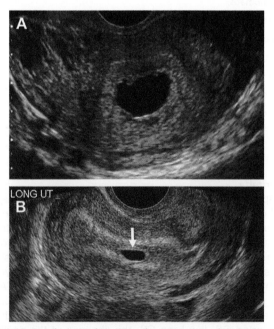

Fig. 7. Abnormal gestational sac in the pre embryonic stage. (*A*) A transverse TVUS image demonstrates a large, irregular intrauterine gestational sac without an embryo. (*B*) A sagittal TVUS image shows a low implantation of intrauterine gestational sac (*arrow*).

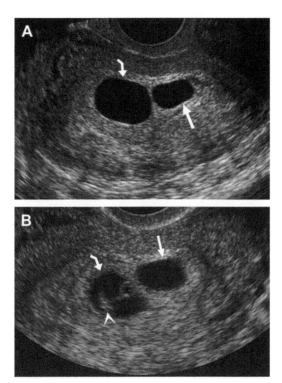

Fig. 8. Anembryonic gestation. (*A*) TVUS demonstrates at 4-weeks menstrual age demonstrates two intrauterine gestational sacs (*arrows*). (*B*) Follow up TVUS after 2 weeks demonstrates a yolk sac and embryo (*arrowhead*) in one gestational sac (*curved arrow*) and anembryonic second gestational sac (*arrow*).

shape, size, and appearance of YS is a sequela of early embryonic demise rather than its cause.[34] An echogenic YS has also been associated with aneuploidy.[35] However, the significance of YS in predicting the pregnancy outcome is uncertain and follow up US is recommended.[36,37]

Embryonic Stage

Once an embryo is identified in the GS, documentation of embryonic cardiac activity is the primary criterion for assessment of pregnancy viability. Though cardiac activity can be identified in embryos as small as 2 mm, the accepted standard CRL at which cardiac activity should be identified is 5 mm.[26] An embryo with a CRL of 5 mm or greater without cardiac activity is a definite sign of nonviable gestation.[18] Embryos with CRL less than 5 mm without cardiac activity should undergo follow-up US.[19] Embryonic bradycardia and small sac size are poor prognostic signs in a viable embryo with cardiac activity. Embryonic bradycardia is defined as a heart rate less than 100 bpm before 6.3 weeks and less than 120 bpm between 6.3 weeks and 7.0 weeks of gestation.[38,39] The relationship of the GS size to the embryo is an important prognostic feature. A difference of less than 5 mm between the mean GS diameter and CRL of embryo is associated with high incidence of abortion. This is called "small sac syndrome" or oligohydramnios (**Fig. 10**).[14,40] A follow up US is recommended in

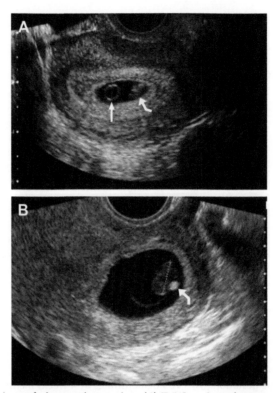

Fig. 9. Yolk sac signs of abnormal gestation. (*A*) TVUS at 6-weeks menstrual age demonstrates an intrauterine gestational sac with an embryo (*curved arrow*) and an abnormally large yolk sac (*arrow*). (*B*) TVUS of another patient at 7 weeks shows an intrauterine gestational sac with embryo and an echogenic yolk sac (*curved arrow*). Both patients eventually had complete abortion.

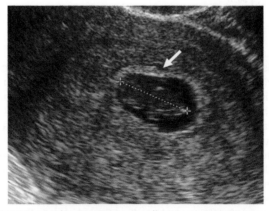

Fig. 10. Coronal TVUS image demonstrates a small intrauterine gestational sac (*arrow*) with an embryo (*cursors*). The difference between mean sac diameter and CRL is less than 5 mm. Follow-up US revealed embryonic demise.

embryonic bradycardia and if there is a discrepancy between the CRL and mean GS diameter.

Anatomic Factors in Spontaneous Abortion

Anatomic uterine defects are associated with about 15% of recurrent spontaneous abortions.[41] These uterine abnormalities are because of congenital mullerian duct fusion anomalies, such as septate or bicornuate uterus, and acquired causes, such as uterine leiomyomas, intrauterine adhesions, and polyps. Recurrent abortions in a septate and bicornuate uterus are because of reduced intrauterine volume or from inadequate vascularity (**Fig. 11**).[42,43] The outcome of pregnancy in the presence of uterine leiomyomas depends upon their size, number, location, and relationship to the placenta. Large submucosal, and multiple and retroplacental leiomyomas are associated with spontaneous abortion (**Fig. 12**).[44–46] Pregnancy associated with an intrauterine contraceptive device (IUCD) in situ is another acquired cause of vaginal bleeding and spontaneous abortion. US is useful to identify the IUCD and its relationship to the GS. The IUCD is extra-amniotic and generally away from the implantation site. Removal of an IUCD in the first trimester increases the chances of continuing a pregnancy to term (**Fig. 13**).[47–49]

Subchorionic Hemorrhage

Approximately 18% to 20% of women presenting with first trimester bleeding have sonographic evidence of subchorionic hematoma. They appear as extrachorionic crescentic anechoic or complex collection, with acute hematomas being

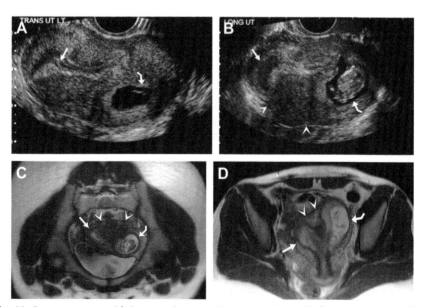

Fig. 11. Septate uterus with intrauterine gestation presenting with first trimester bleeding. TVUS images (*A, B*) demonstrate two separate endometrial cavities with gestational sac and embryo (*curved arrow*) in one endometrial cavity and decidual reaction with fluid in another endometrial cavity (*arrow*). Corresponding coronal (*C*) and axial (*D*) T2-weighted images of the pelvis confirm the septate uterus with intrauterine gestation in one endometrial cavity (*curved arrow*). The intervening septum (*arrowheads*) is demonstrated in both TVUS and MR images.

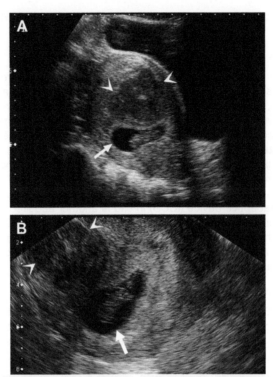

Fig. 12. Fibroid uterus with first trimester bleeding. Transabdominal (*A*) and TVUS (*B*) sagittal images demonstrate a fibroid in the ventral myometrial wall (*arrowheads*) deforming the intrauterine gestational sac with embryo (*arrow*). The pregnancy continued to term without complications.

more echogenic (**Fig. 14**). The size of the hematoma can be measured by either volume or by the percentage of chorionic sac circumference elevated by the hematoma. There are variable reports regarding the outcome of pregnancy in patients with subchorionic hematoma.[50–55] The outcome depends upon the size of the hematoma, gestational age, and maternal age. The outcome is generally poor with large hematomas in women over age 35 presenting before 8 weeks of gestation.[50–52,55]

Retained Products of Conception

Patients presenting with persistent bleeding following spontaneous abortion undergo TVUS for detection of retained products of conception. Retained products of conception are associated with an increased risk of bleeding and infection, and delayed complications, such as disseminated intravascular coagulation and infertility because of endometrial osseous metaplasia.[56] The appearance of retained products of conception is highly variable. A GS with a nonviable embryo or an irregular GS may be identified. Any endometrial mass or complex fluid collection irrespective of vascularity on Doppler evaluation should be considered as retained products of conception.[56,57] Color flow and pulsed Doppler is useful in identification of retained trophoblastic tissue, as it demonstrates low-resistance arterial flow (**Fig. 15**). A thick endometrial lining of more than 10 mm is a less sensitive sign of retained products

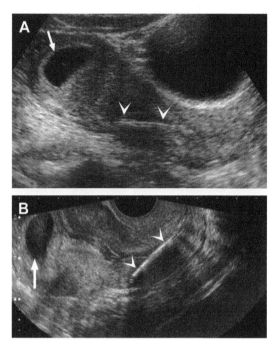

Fig. 13. Intrauterine pregnancy in a misplaced IUCD presenting with first trimester bleeding. Transabdominal (*A*) and TVUS (*B*) sagittal images demonstrate a low IUCD (*arrowheads*) with its tip extending into the posterior myometrial wall and an early intrauterine gestational sac (*arrow*). Follow-up TVUS after removal of the IUCD confirmed dichorionic diamniotic twin intrauterine gestation.

and should be correlated with clinical presentation and serial quantitative beta hCG.[58,59] The retained products of conception are occasionally identified either in the endocervical canal or vagina, indicating an abortion in progress (**Fig. 16**).

UTERINE ARTERIOVENOUS MALFORMATIONS

Uterine AVMs were first described by Dubriel and Loubat in 1926.[60] They are either congenital or acquired in nature and are an uncommon but a potentially life threatening cause of vaginal bleeding. They are rarely associated with first trimester bleeding and spontaneous abortion. Congenital vascular malformations result from arrested vascular development and are composed of multiple vascular channels of variable caliber with fistulous communications within the myometrium. The acquired AVMs are the result of arteriovenous fistula between a single artery and single vein. The acquired arteriovenous fistulae result from previous trauma, infection, or malignancy. Previous trauma can be from abortion, dilation, and curettage, cesarian section, or IUCD. The malignant causes include cervical carcinoma, endometrial carcinoma, and gestational trophoblastic.[61,62]

Sonographic Features of Arteriovenous Malformations

The gray scale US features of AVM are variable. The most common finding is a spongy appearance of the myometrium because of multiple tubular and cystic anechoic

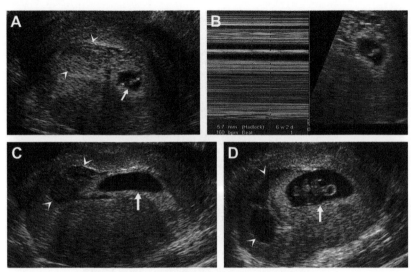

Fig. 14. Subchorionic hemorrhage. (*A*) Coronal TVUS image demonstrates an intrauterine gestational sac (*arrow*) with embryo (*cursors*) and an echogenic acute subchorionic hemorrhage (*arrowheads*). (*B*) Cardiac activity with a heart rate of 160 bpm is recorded. Follow-up TVUS after 2 weeks (*C*) demonstrates decrease in the echotexture of the hematoma (*arrowheads*) and after 4 weeks (*D*) demonstrates normal progression of the gestational sac and embryo (*arrow*) with a stable more anechoic subchorionic hematoma (*arrowheads*).

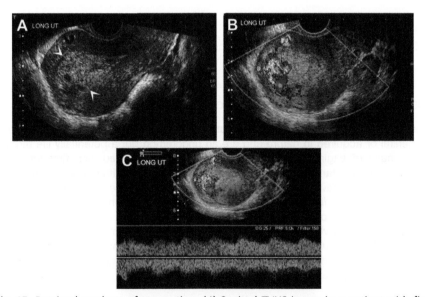

Fig. 15. Retained products of conception. (*A*) Sagittal TVUS image in a patient with first trimester vaginal bleeding demonstrates heterogeneous intrauterine contents (*arrowheads*) without a definite gestational sac. Color flow Doppler (*B*) shows increased vascularity of the complex endometrial contents and pulsed Doppler (*C*) reveals low resistance arterial flow.

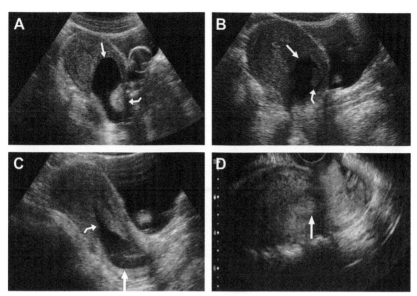

Fig. 16. Abortion in progress. (*A, B*) Transabdominal US images demonstrate a low-lying gestational sac (*arrow*) with trophoblastic tissue (*curved arrow* in *A*) and embryo (*curved arrow* in *B*). (*C*) Subsequent transabdominal scan shows extension of the products of conception through the internal os (*curved arrow*) into the cervix (*arrow*). (*D*) Final transabdominal US image shows a collapsed endocervical canal (*arrow*) after complete expulsion of the products of conception.

spaces (**Fig. 17**A). They may occasionally present as a focal myometrial mass resembling a fibroid. A polypoidal endometrial mass may be present.[62]

Color flow Doppler for AVM demonstrates a mosaic pattern color signal within the cystic spaces (**Fig. 17**B). Spectral analysis of these vascular spaces demonstrates high velocity and low resistance flow in the arteries, and pulsatile high velocity venous flow (**Fig. 17**C). Large AVMs are associated with prominent parametrial vessels.[60–62] There is considerable overlap of US features of AVM with those of retained products of conception following a spontaneous abortion and gestational trophoblastic disease (GTD).[10,63] Correlation with serum quantitative beta hCG is important to differentiate AVM from these two entities. This differentiation is crucial as management of an AVM by dilatation and curettage (see 17 D and C) can be catastrophic. MR imaging with intravenous gadolinium is useful in large congenital AVMs to assess the extent of myometrial and parametrial involvement.[62] Management of AVM is by selective arterial embolization and hysterectomy. An acquired AVM fistula is more amenable for arterial embolization because of a single or few feeding arteries.[60,61,64,65]

ECTOPIC PREGNANCY

Ectopic pregnancy remains an important cause of maternal mortality, accounting for 9% of all pregnancy-related deaths in 1992. The incidence of ectopic pregnancy has increased from 4.5 per 1,000 pregnancies in 1970 to 19.7 per 1,000 pregnancies in 1992.[66] This increased incidence is partly because of additional risk factors, but mostly the result of improvement in diagnostic methods. Ectopic pregnancy is defined as implantation of the fertilized ovum outside the uterine cavity. Approximately 97% of

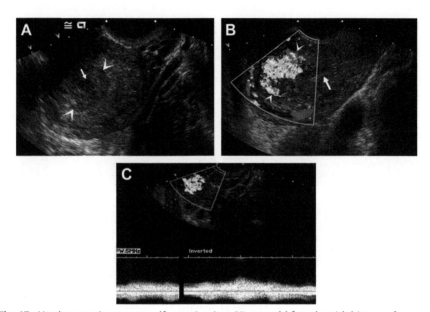

Fig. 17. Uterine arteriovenous malformation in a 35-year-old female with history of sponta-neous abortion presenting with vaginal bleeding. She was referred to exclude retained products of conception. (*A*) TVUS shows a complex myometrial mass (*arrowheads*) with anechoic spaces (*arrow*). (*B*) Corresponding color flow Doppler demonstrates the mosaic pattern of flow within the mass (*arrowheads*). Arrow points to the collapsed endometrial cavity. (*C*) Pulsed Doppler demonstrates arterialized venous flow diagnostic of arteriovenous malformation.

ectopic pregnancies occur in the fallopian tube and the remaining 3% occur in the cervix, ovary, or abdominal cavity. Ampulla is the most common site of tubal preg-nancy, seen in 55% of all tubal pregnancies. The isthmus and fimbrial ends are less common sites of tubal pregnancy, accounting for 25% and 17%, respectively (**Fig. 18**).[67] The risk factors for ectopic pregnancy include pelvic inflammatory disease, previous ectopic pregnancy, endometriosis, previous tubal surgery, uterotubal anom-alies, in utero exposure to diethylstilbestrol, and cigarette smoking.[68,69] Previous ectopic pregnancy is a significant risk factor, with a recurrence rate of 15% to 20% following treatment of an ectopic pregnancy.[70–72] Abdominal pain and vaginal

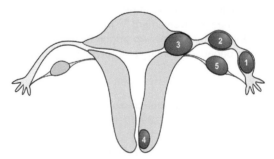

Fig. 18. Line diagram illustrates the various locations of ectopic pregnancy: (**1**) ampulla (**2**) isthmus (**3**) interstitial (**4**) cervix (**5**) ovary.

bleeding or spotting with a history of amenorrhea is the most common presentation of ectopic pregnancy. This presentation is nonspecific and can be seen with threatened or spontaneous abortion. More specific signs are localized adnexal pain and tenderness, peritoneal signs with pain radiating to the shoulder, and hypovolemic shock are less commonly seen. Therefore, a high index of clinical suspicion and diagnostic workup with serum beta hCG and US is the key to the early diagnosis of ectopic pregnancy.

Sonographic Features of Ectopic Pregnancy

A summary of sonographic findings of ectopic pregnancy is shown in **Table 3**. When the serum beta hCG is above the discriminatory level of 1,500 IU and no intrauterine GS is identified, a careful search of the adnexa with TVUS is mandatory for an extrauterine GS.[4,6] In the absence of an intrauterine GS associated with serum beta hCG below the discriminatory level, follow-up with serial quantitative beta hCG and US is necessary until a conclusive diagnosis is made.[25] A pseudogestational sac is seen in 10% to 20% of ectopic pregnancies because of decidual reaction of the endometrial lining and fluid in the endometrial cavity (**Fig. 19**A, **Fig. 20**A). Differentiation from a true GS is made by absence of "double decidual sac" sign and presence of a YS or embryo.[5,6,73] The most common sonographic finding is an extra ovarian complex adnexal mass with or without free fluid in the pelvis.[67,74] This adnexal mass is because of a combination of a dilated fallopian tube with a GS, with or without a hematosalpinx and surrounding hematoma (see **Fig. 19**). This extra ovarian adnexal mass has a sensitivity of 84.4%, specificity of 98.9%, and positive predictive value (PPV) of 96.3%.[73] The appearance of pelvic fluid in addition to the adnexal mass further increases the sensitivity and specificity. The presence of echogenic fluid in the pelvis because of hemoperitoneum has a much higher predictive value, and a moderate amount of echogenic fluid in the pelvis can be an isolated finding of an ectopic pregnancy.[75] The echogenic fluid in the pelvis represents either tubal abortion or rupture (**Fig. 21**).[76] The most definitive sign of ectopic pregnancy is the demonstration of an extrauterine GS with a YS or embryo (see **Fig. 20**). However, a YS and embryo are less commonly seen. The extrauterine GS is most often seen as an empty cystic structure, which has to be differentiated from the more common ovarian corpus luteum cyst. The ectopic GS has a 2-mm to 4-mm thick echogenic rim and represents the tubal ring sign of ectopic pregnancy (**Fig. 22**).[77] The tubal ring of an ectopic gestation is more echogenic than the ovarian parenchyma and the endometrial lining.[78,79] The corpus luteum cyst has a wide range of sonographic appearance and can have a thick echogenic rim similar to the ectopic GS. Color flow Doppler is not useful in

Table 3 Sonographic features of ectopic pregnancy	
Sonographic Signs	**Comments**
Absence of an IUGS with a serum beta hCG above the discriminatory level (1,000 mIU/L)	Evaluation of adnexa for ectopic location of GS
Pseudogestational sac	Absence of a DDS sign
Extraovarian complex adnexal mass	Most common sign
Adnexal tubal ring sign	Mimics an exophytic corpus luteum cyst
Echogenic free fluid	Indicates hemorrhage and may or may not be associated with rupture of the ectopic gestation

Abbreviations: DDS, double decidual sac sign; IUGS, intrauterine gestational sac.

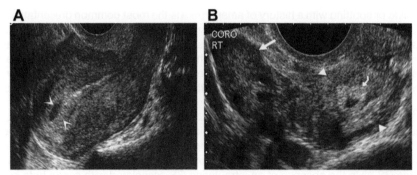

Fig. 19. Ectopic pregnancy. (*A*) Sagittal TVUS of the uterus demonstrates decidual reaction and minimal fluid in the endometrial cavity (*arrowheads*) and no intrauterine gestational sac. (*B*) Coronal TVUS of the right adnexa shows ovary (*arrow*) and an extra ovarian adnexal mass (*arrowheads*) with a gestational sac (*curved arrow*).

differentiating these two, as both can demonstrate increased vascularity, giving the "ring of fire" appearance.[79,80] Spectral Doppler and measurement of the resistive index (RI) may be useful in differentiating these two. The RI of the corpus luteum cysts is reported to vary from 0.39 to 0.7 and the RI of the ectopic GS is either less than 0.39 or greater than 0.7. This has a reported specificity and PPV of 100% in the diagnosis of ectopic pregnancy.[80] The above described sonographic signs are those seen in the more common tubal ectopic pregnancy. Interstitial, cervical, and ovarian ectopic pregnancies have more distinctive sonographic appearances.

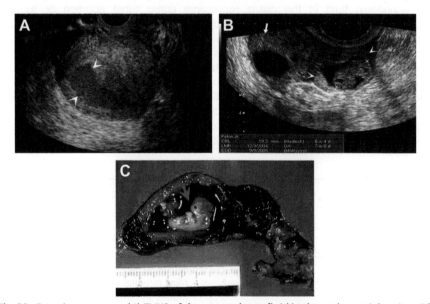

Fig. 20. Ectopic pregnancy. (*A*) TVUS of the uterus shows fluid in the endometrial cavity with thin decidual reaction representing pseudo gestational sac (*arrowheads*). (*B*) TVUS image of the right adnexa demonstrates right ovary (*arrow*) and ectopic tubal gestational sac (*arrowheads*) with an embryo (*cursors*). (*C*) Photograph of the salpingectomy specimen demonstrates a fallopian tube with ectopic gestational sac and an embryo (*arrow*).

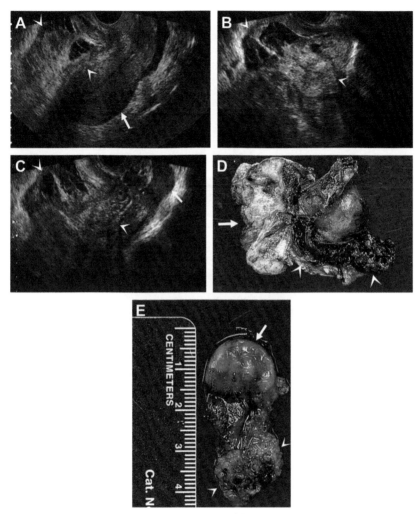

Fig. 21. Ruptured ectopic pregnancy. A 24-year-old, hemodynamically unstable female with positive pregnancy test and severe abdominal pain. (*A*) Sagittal TVUS image shows an empty uterus (*arrow*) and a large complex mass (*arrowheads*) adjacent to the uterus. (*B, C*) TVUS images show complex adnexal mass (*arrowheads*) with mixed anechoic and echogenic components and echogenic free fluid (*arrow*) in the cul-de-sac. No discrete ectopic gestational sac is identified. (*D*) Photograph of the gross specimen shows ruptured fallopian tube with hematosalpinx (*arrowheads*) and the adjacent ovary (*arrow*). (*E*) Gross specimen photograph of the extracted embryo (*arrow*) and the trophoblastic tissue (*arrowheads*).

Interstitial Pregnancy

The interstitial segment of the fallopian tube is the proximal portion of the tube that is within the myometrial wall of the uterus (see **Fig. 18**). It is about 1 cm to 2 cm in length and 0.7-mm wide. It is highly vascular because of the combined vascular supply from the uterine and ovarian vessels. Interstitial pregnancy is a rare type of ectopic pregnancy, accounting for 2% to 4% of all tubal pregnancies, but has high maternal mortality because of catastrophic hemorrhage. The high vascularity of this region

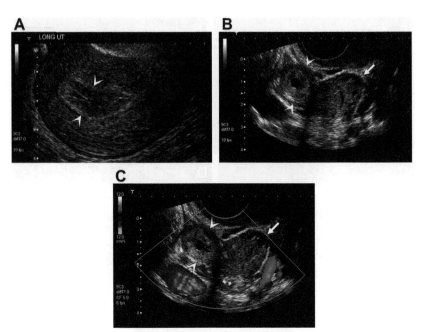

Fig. 22. Tubal ring sign of ectopic pregnancy. (*A*) Sagittal TVUS of the uterus demonstrates minimal fluid in the endometrial cavity with surrounding decidual reaction (*arrowheads*) representing a pseudogestational sac. (*B, C*) Gray scale and color flow Doppler TVUS images of the right adnexa show ovary (*arrow*) and an extra ovarian anechoic focus with surrounding thick echogenic rim (*arrowheads*) representing the "tubal ring sign" of an early ectopic tubal gestation.

and delayed rupture because of the surrounding protective myometrial wall are responsible for the high mortality of these patients. The ultrasound findings include an eccentric GS near the uterine cornual region with surrounding myometrial mantle. The surrounding myometrial mantle is thin, incomplete, and is generally 5-mm thick (**Fig. 23**).[81–83] The "interstitial line" sign, because of a linear echogenic endometrial lining extending to the edge of the eccentric GS, is reported to be highly sensitive and specific for the diagnosis of interstitial ectopic pregnancy (**Fig. 24**). The interstitial line sign has a sensitivity of 80% and specificity of 98% as compared with eccentric GS location (sensitivity, 40%; specificity, 88%) and thin myometrial mantle (sensitivity, 40%; specificity, 93%) for the diagnosis of interstitial pregnancy.[84] An eccentric location of intrauterine GS because of uterine contraction, uterine leiomyomas, or a GS within the horn of a bicornuate uterus can mimic an interstitial ectopic pregnancy. Angular pregnancy is an intrauterine pregnancy in the lateral angle of the uterine cavity medial to the uterotubal junction, and can be mistaken for an interstitial ectopic gestation because of eccentric position of the GS.[85,86] Three-dimensional US and MR imaging may be used when two-dimensional US findings of interstitial pregnancy are equivocal.[87–90]

Ovarian Pregnancy

Ovarian pregnancy is an uncommon ectopic pregnancy with a reported incidence varying from 1 in 6,000 to 1 in 40,000 pregnancies.[91] The ratio of ovarian pregnancy

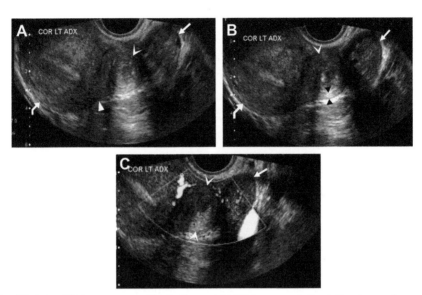

Fig. 23. Interstitial pregnancy. (*A, B*) Coronal TVUS images of the left adnexa show an ectopic gestational sac (*arrowhead*) between the left ovary (*arrow*) and uterus (*curved arrow*) with myometrial extension (*solid arrowhead*) and myometrial mantle (*black arrowheads*) surrounding the gestational sac. (*C*) Corresponding color flow Doppler image demonstrates combined ovarian and uterine vascular supply to the ectopic gestation.

to all other ectopic pregnancies is 1% to 6%.[92] There are few reports of multiple ovarian gestations.[92,93] The risk factors for ovarian pregnancy are similar to those of tubal pregnancy, which include pelvic inflammatory disease, IUCD usage, previous surgery, and endometriosis.[92–94] Spiegelberg in 1878 set four criteria for the diagnosis of ovarian pregnancy: normal tube on the affected side, GS located at the anatomic site of the ovary, GS connected to the uterus by the utero-ovarian ligament, and ovarian tissue demonstrated in the GS wall.[95] The GS may be within the substance of the ovary or on its surface and will appear as an echogenic ring with central sonolucent area (**Fig. 25**). In the absence of a YS and embryo, it may be mistaken for

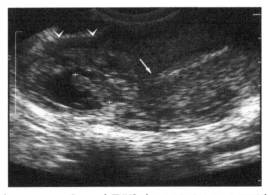

Fig. 24. Interstitial pregnancy. Coronal TVUS demonstrates an eccentric right interstitial gestational sac with embryo (*within calipers*). The endometrial lining extending to the edge of the gestational sac, "interstitial line" sign (*arrow*) and the surrounding myometrial mantle (*arrowheads*) are well demonstrated.

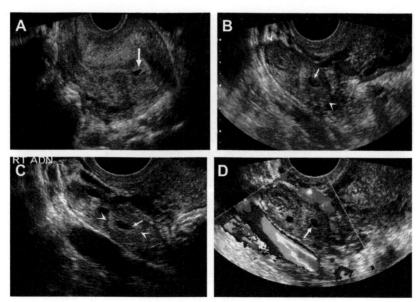

Fig. 25. Ovarian pregnancy. A patient with positive pregnancy test and a serum beta hCG of 1,200 IU presents with pelvic pain and vaginal spotting. (*A*) Sagittal TVUS of the uterus shows a pseudo gestational sac (*arrow*). (*B*) TVUS image of the right adnexa shows a small anechoic focus with thick echogenic wall (*arrow*) within the right ovary (*arrowheads*). No other adnexal mass was identified. Patient had curettage of the endometrial contents, which revealed decidual reaction and no chorionic tissue. (*C*) Follow-up TVUS because of persistent elevation of beta hCG revealed persistent suspicious gestational sac (*arrowheads*) within the right ovary with suggestion of a yolk sac (*arrow*). (*D*) Corresponding color flow Doppler TVUS image of the right ovary with suspicious gestational sac (*arrow*). Laparoscopic surgery and pathology confirmed ectopic right ovarian gestation.

a hemorrhagic cyst on both TVUS and at surgery.[96–98] The diagnosis in such cases is usually made by the pathologist.[97] The risk of rupture and hemorrhage in ovarian pregnancy is similar to tubal pregnancy.

Cervical Pregnancy

Cervical pregnancy is an uncommon intrauterine ectopic pregnancy caused by implantation of the GS in the endocervical canal. It is potentially life threatening because of the increased risk of bleeding.[99] It has to be differentiated from the more common products of conception in the cervical canal during spontaneous abortion. The GS of a cervical pregnancy is round or oval and may demonstrate a YS or an embryo (**Fig. 26**). The GS in the products of conception during an abortion is collapsed and crenated.[100–102] Demonstration of trophoblastic flow in the cervix by color Doppler is more suggestive of a cervical pregnancy. There is always some evidence of decidual reaction or hemorrhagic products in the endometrial cavity with an open internal os of the cervix in patients with abortion in progress (see **Fig. 16**). A sliding motion of the GS against the cervical canal by gentle pressure with the endovaginal probe described as the "sliding sign" is seen in spontaneous abortion, where as the GS is fixed in cervical pregnancy.[103] There are reports of potential advantages of MR imaging in the diagnosis of cervical pregnancy, when US findings are inconclusive.[104,105]

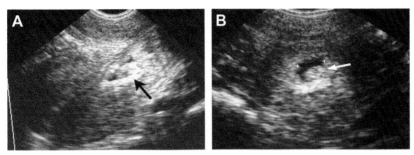

Fig. 26. Cervical pregnancy. Sagittal (*A*) and coronal (*B*) TVUS images of the uterus demonstrate a gestational sac with embryo (*arrow*) implanted within the cervix.

Management of Ectopic Pregnancy

There are several treatment options for ectopic pregnancy, including expectant treatment, systemic methotrexate injection, US-guided local injection of methotrexate or potassium chloride, and surgery. Surgical management can be either a salpingectomy or a salpingostomy with preservation of the tube. The criteria for medical management include a hemodynamically stable patient who is compliant for posttreatment follow-up, pretreatment beta hCG of greater than 5,000 IU and the absence of embryonic cardiac activity.[106,107] After the first injection of methotrexate, weekly serum beta hCG follow-up is mandatory. A second dose of methotrexate is administered if there is less than a 15% decline in the serum beta hCG.[108–110] Cervical, interstitial, and cesarean scar pregnancies may be treated by US-guided local injection of methotrexate or potassium chloride.[111]

GESTATIONAL TROPHOBLASTIC DISEASE

GTD encompasses a spectrum of conditions derived from the placental trophoblasts, including hydatidiform mole, invasive mole, choriocarcinoma, and placental site trophoblastic tumor. GTD is characterized by abnormal proliferation of the trophoblastic tissue with varying degree of malignant potential and increased beta hCG production.[112,113] Classification of GTD is displayed in **Box 2**.

Hydatidiform Mole

The incidence of molar pregnancy is higher in Asian countries than in the United States and Europe. The reported incidence of molar pregnancy in the United States is 1 in

---

Box 2
Classification of gestational trophoblastic disease

Hydatidiform mole

    Partial mole

    Complete mole

Gestational trophoblastic neoplasia

    Invasive mole

    Choriocarcinoma

    Placental site trophoblastic tumor

1,000 deliveries. The incidence of molar pregnancy is also higher in teenage women and after age 35.[114–116] Maternal age and previous molar pregnancy are the two major risk factors. The hydatidiform mole is classified into complete molar pregnancy and partial molar pregnancy, based on the absence or presence of a fetus. The complete molar pregnancy has no fetus and partial molar pregnancy is associated with a fetus. Both types are characterized by abnormal proliferation of trophoblastic cells and hydropic villi. The karyotype in a complete mole is 46XX, with both chromosomes of paternal origin, and is referred to as "androgenesis." The karyotype of a partial mole is triploid (69, XXY) or even tetraploid (92, XXXY), with one paternal chromosome and the rest of maternal origin.[117,118] A complete mole is a result of fertilization of a defective ovum by a sperm and all chromosomes are derived from the sperm.

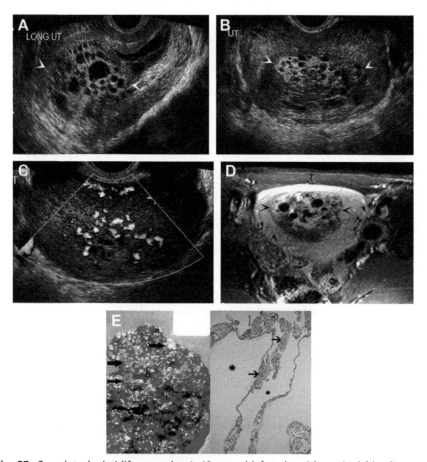

Fig. 27. Complete hydatidiform mole. A 40-year-old female with vaginal bleeding and a serum beta hCG of 200,000 mIU/mL. Sagittal (A) and coronal (B) TVUS images of the uterus show a complex mass (*arrowheads*) with multiple anechoic cystic foci corresponding to hydropic villi of molar pregnancy. There is no associated embryo. (C) Coronal TVUS with power Doppler demonstrates typical trophoblastic flow within the mass. (D) Corresponding T1-weighted postgadolinium axial image of the uterus demonstrates multiple well-defined hypointense lesions representing the hydropic villi of molar pregnancy. (E) Specimen photograph shows cystic villi (*arrows*) and photomicrograph shows hydropic villi (*flowers*) and trophoblastic hyperplasia (*arrows*).

The gross appearance of a complete mole consists of a cluster of edematous vesicles 5 mm to 2 cm in size and in varying degrees of hemorrhage and necrosis.[119] The clinical presentation of molar pregnancy in the early first trimester is indistinguishable from a normal pregnancy or a threatened abortion. The classic presentation of vaginal bleeding, enlarged uterus, absent fetal tone, and hyperemesis are seen in the late first trimester and second trimester of pregnancy. Pregnancy-induced hypertension before 20 weeks and thyrotoxicosis are other clinical presentations. Serum beta hCG levels are elevated and are usually over 100,000 mIU/mL. Serum beta hCG levels are higher in complete mole than in partial mole. Because of the regular practice of first trimester US, molar pregnancy is diagnosed by US before the patient has typical clinical presentation.[120]

Sonographic Features of Molar Pregnancy

TVUS is the imaging modality for the diagnosis and follow up of molar pregnancy. The sonographic appearance is variable and depends upon the size of the vesicles, associated hemorrhage, and necrosis. The classic appearance is a mass in the endometrial cavity composed of multiple cystic anechoic spaces, which vary in size from 1 mm to 30 mm. The size of the cystic spaces is larger with advancing gestational age. The mass appears more echogenic and solid with small cystic spaces.[121,122] Color flow Doppler demonstrates some of the cystic spaces to be vascular with a high velocity and low resistance flow (**Fig. 27**). The degree of invasion of the myometrium by the molar tissue is variable. Doppler evaluation improves the accuracy of the depth of myometrial invasion by the molar tissue.[123,124] Comparing the sonographic features with serum beta hCG is useful to differentiate molar pregnancy from retained products of conception and blood clots in a patient with spontaneous abortion. Retained trophoblastic tissue with hydropic degeneration closely resembles molar pregnancy on US. Increased myometrial involvement is a feature of molar pregnancy and myometrial invasion of more than one-third of its depth is useful in differentiating molar pregnancy from retained products of conception.[125] In a partial molar pregnancy, a GS with an embryo is seen in addition to the molar tissue (**Fig. 28**). About 25% to 60% of cases with molar pregnancy have thecaleutin cysts because of hyperstimulation of the ovaries by the increased hCG. The ovaries are enlarged, with multiple cysts replacing the entire ovary, and have a "soap bubble" or "spoke-wheel" appearance (**Fig. 29**).[121,126]

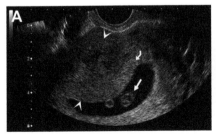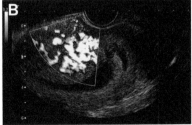

Fig. 28. Partial mole. A 35-year-old female with past history of molar pregnancy, presenting with hyperemesis and a serum beta hCG of 185,000 mIU/mL. (*A*) TVUS of the uterus shows an intrauterine gestational sac (*curved arrow*) with an embryo (*straight arrow*). A complex mass (*arrowheads*) with multiple anechoic foci in the myometrium corresponds to an associated hydatidiform mole. (*B*) TVUS with power Doppler demonstrates typical trophoblastic flow within the complex mass.

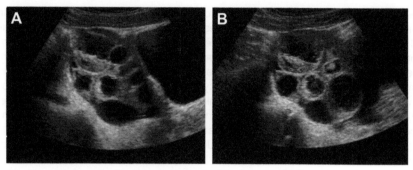

Fig. 29. Thecaleutin cysts. (*A, B*) Transabdominal US images of bilateral ovaries in a patient with molar pregnancy demonstrates enlarged ovaries with multiple cysts of varying sizes.

Gestational Trophoblastic Neoplasia

Gestational trophoblastic neoplasia (GTN) includes invasive molar pregnancy and choriocarcinoma. The invasive mole is characterized by local invasion of the myometrium without distant hematogeneous metastases (**Fig. 30**). The choriocarcinoma is a malignant form of molar pregnancy, with distant hematogenous metastases to the lungs, liver, brain, and other organs. MR imaging is more accurate in demonstrating the depth of myometrial invasion by the molar tissue than US. The distant metastases

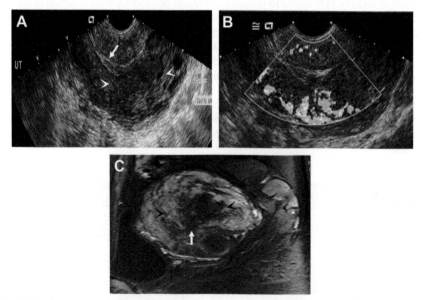

Fig. 30. Invasive mole. Follow-up ultrasonography in a patient for persistent elevation of serum beta hCG following evacuation of a complete hydatidiform mole. (*A*) Sagittal TVUS of the uterus demonstrates an illdefined mass (*arrowheads*) in the myometrium extending from the endometrial cavity (*arrow*). (*B*) Corresponding color Doppler image of the uterus shows vascularity of the infiltrating myometrial mass. (*C*) Axial postgadolinium T1-weighted image of the uterus demonstrates endometrial cavity (*arrow*) and the infiltrating mass in the myometrium (*black arrowheads*).

in choriocarcinoma are better evaluated by CT scan. Choriocarcinoma is preceded by hydatidiform mole in 50% of cases, spontaneous abortion in 25%, normal pregnancy in 22.5%, and ectopic pregnancy in 2.5%. Choriocarcinoma is suspected in all patients with persistent elevation of serum beta hCG after evacuation of a molar pregnancy.[121,122,127]

SUMMARY

First trimester vaginal bleeding is a common clinical presentation to the emergency department. Clinical assessment of the viability of the pregnancy is unreliable at this early stage of pregnancy. TVUS is an essential imaging modality to confirm an intra-uterine gestation and a living embryo. Knowledge of the normal sonographic mile-stones of early intrauterine gestation helps differentiate a normal from abnormal intrauterine gestation in the pre-embryonic stage and a pseudogestational sac of ectopic pregnancy from a true intrauterine GS. TVUS also plays a crucial role in the diagnosis of ectopic gestation and its suitability for conservative management. Follow-up of postabortion patients with persistent bleeding is performed with TVUS to identify retained products of conception. TVUS is also useful to identify rare causes of first trimester bleeding, such as GTD and AVM of the uterus.

ACKNOWLEDGMENTS

The authors thank Joseph Molter for his assistance in preparation of figures for this article.

REFERENCES

1. Nyberg DA, Laing FC, Filly RA. Threatened abortion: sonographic distinction of normal and abnormal gestation sacs. Radiology 1986;158:397–400.
2. Barnhart KT, Simhan H, Kamelle SA. Diagnostic accuracy of ultrasound above and below the beta-hCG discriminatory zone. Obstet Gynecol 1999;94:583–7.
3. Nyberg DA, Filly RA, Mahony BS, et al. Early gestation: correlation of HCG levels and sonographic identification. AJR Am J Roentgenol 1985;144:951–4.
4. Banhart K, Mennuti MT, Benjamin I, et al. Prompt diagnosis of ectopic pregnancy in an emergency department setting. Obstet Gynecol 1994;84:1010–5.
5. Bradley WG, Fiske CE, Filly RA. The double sac sign of early intrauterine pregnancy: use in exclusion of ectopic pregnancy. Radiology 1982;143:223–6.
6. Mahony BS, Filly RA, Nyberg DA, et al. Sonographic evaluation of ectopic pregnancy. J Ultrasound Med 1985;4:221–8.
7. Levi CS, Lyons EA, Lindsay DJ. Early diagnosis of nonviable pregnancy with transvaginal US. Radiology 1988;167:383–5.
8. Nyberg DA, Mack LA, Harvey D, et al. Value of the yolk sac in evaluating early pregnancies. J Ultrasound Med 1988;7:129–35.
9. Wiebe ER, Switzer P. Arteriovenous malformations of the uterus associated with medical abortion. Int J Gynaecol Obstet 2000;71:155–8.
10. Kido A, Togashi K, Koyama T, et al. Retained products of conception masquerading as acquired arteriovenous malformation. J Comput Assist Tomogr 2003;27:88–92.
11. Implementation of the principle of as low as reasonably achievable (ALARA) for medical and dental personnel. NRCP report 107. Bethesda (MD): National Council on Radiation Protection and Measurements; 1990.

12. Emerson DS, Cartier MS, Altieri LA, et al. Diagnostic efficacy of endovaginal color flow imaging in an ectopic pregnancy screening program. Radiology 1992;183:413–20.

13. Yeh HC, Goodman JD, Carr L, et al. Intradecidual sign: a US criterion of early intrauterine pregnancy. Radiology 1986;161:463–7.

14. Rowling SE, Coleman BG, Langer JE, et al. First-trimester US parameters of failed pregnancy. Radiology 1997;203:211–7.

15. Coulam CB, Britten S, Soenksen DM. Early (34–56 days from last menstrual period) ultrasonographic measurements in normal pregnancies. Hum Reprod 1996;11:1771–4.

16. Goldstein SR, Wolfson R. Transvaginal ultrasonographic measurement of early embryonic size as a means of assessing gestational age. J Ultrasound Med 1994;13:27–31.

17. Wisser J, Dirschedl P, Krone S. Estimation of gestational age by transvaginal sonographic measurement of the greatest embryonic length in dated human embryos. Ultrasound Obstet Gynecol 1994;4:457–62.

18. Goldstein SR. Significance of cardiac activity on endovaginal ultrasound in very early embryos. Obstet Gynecol 1992;80:670–2.

19. Levi CS, Lyons EA, Zheng XH, et al. Endovaginal US: demonstration of cardiac activity in embryos of less than 5.0 mm in crown rump length. Radiology 1990; 176:71–4.

20. Hertzberg BS, Mahony BS, Bowie JD. First trimester fetal cardiac activity. Sonographic documentation of a progressive early rise in heart rate. J Ultrasound Med 1988;7:573–5.

21. Yeh HC, Rabinowitz JG. Amniotic sac development: ultrasound features of early pregnancy—the double bleb sign. Radiology 1988;166(1 Pt 1):97–103.

22. Ulm B, Ulm MR, Bernaschek G. Unfused amnion and chorion after 14 weeks of gestation: associated fetal structural and chromosomal abnormalities. Ultrasound Obstet Gynecol 1999;13:392–5.

23. Bromley B, Shipp TD, Benacerraf BR. Amnion-chorion separation after 17 weeks' gestation. Obstet Gynecol 1999;94:1024–6.

24. Ljunger E, Cnattingius S, Lundin C, et al. Chromosomal anomalies in first-trimester miscarriages. Acta Obstet Gynecol Scand 2005;84:1103–7.

25. Condous G, Kirk E, Lu C, et al. Diagnostic accuracy of varying discriminatory zones for the prediction of ectopic pregnancy in women with a pregnancy of unknown location. Ultrasound Obstet Gynecol 2005;26:770–5.

26. Levi CS, Lyons EA, Lindsay DJ. Ultrasound in the first trimester of pregnancy. Radiol Clin North Am 1990;28:19–38.

27. Bernard KG, Cooperberg PL. Sonographic differentiation between blighted ovum and early viable pregnancy. AJR Am J Roentgenol 1985;144: 597–602.

28. McKenna KM, Feldstein VA, Goldstein RB, et al. The empty amnion: a sign of early pregnancy failure. J Ultrasound Med 1995;14:117–21.

29. Nyberg DA, Mack LA, Laing FC, et al. Distinguishing normal from abnormal gestational sac growth in early pregnancy. J Ultrasound Med 1987;6:23–7.

30. Levi CS. Prediction of early pregnancy failure on the basis of mean gestational sac size and absence of a sonographically demonstrable yolk sac. Radiology 1995;195:873.

31. Lindsay DJ, Lovett IS, Lyons EA, et al. Yolk sac diameter and shape at endovaginal US: predictors of pregnancy outcome in the first trimester. Radiology 1992; 183:115–8.

32. Stampone C, Nicotra M, Muttinelli C, et al. Transvaginal sonography of the yolk sac in normal and abnormal pregnancy. J Clin Ultrasound 1996;24:3–9.
33. Harris RD, Vincent LM, Askin FB. Yolk sac calcification: a sonographic finding associated with intrauterine embryonic demise in the first trimester. Radiology 1988;166:109–10.
34. Jauniaux E, Jurkovic D, Henriet Y, et al. Development of the secondary human yolk sac: correlation of sonographic and anatomical features. Hum Reprod 1991;6:1160–6.
35. Szabo J, Gellen J, Szemere G, et al. Significance of hyper-echogenic yolk sac in first-trimester screening for chromosome aneuploidy. Orv Hetil 1996;137:2313–5.
36. Reece EA, Scioscia AL, Pinter E, et al. Prognostic significance of the human yolk sac assessed by ultrasonography. Am J Obstet Gynecol 1988;159:1191–4.
37. Kurtz AB, Needleman L, Pennell RG, et al. Can detection of the yolk sac in the first trimester be used to predict the outcome of pregnancy? A prospective sonographic study. AJR Am J Roentgenol 1992;158:843–7.
38. Laboda LA, Estroff JA, Benacerraf BR. First trimester bradycardia. A sign of impending fetal loss. J Ultrasound Med 1989;8:561–3.
39. Doubilet PM, Benson CB. Outcome of first-trimester pregnancies with slow embryonic heart rate at 6–7 weeks gestation and normal heart rate by 8 weeks at US. Radiology 2005;236:643–6.
40. Bromley B, Harlow BL, Laboda LA, et al. Small sac size in the first trimester: a predictor of poor fetal out come. Radiology 1991;178:375–7.
41. Devi Wold AS, Pham N, Arici A. Anatomic factors in recurrent pregnancy loss. Semin Reprod Med 2006;24:25–32.
42. Propst AM, Hill JA 3rd. Anatomic factors associated with recurrent pregnancy loss. Semin Reprod Med 2000;18:341–50.
43. Raga F, Bauset C, Remohi J, et al. Reproductive impact of congenital mullerian anomalies. Hum Reprod 1997;12:2277–81.
44. Benson CB, Chow JS, Chang-Lee W, et al. Outcome of pregnancies in women with uterine leiomyomas identified by sonography in the first trimester. J Clin Ultrasound 2001;29:261–4.
45. Ouyang DW, Economy KE, Norwitz ER. Obstetric complications of fibroids. Obstet Gynecol Clin North Am 2006;33:153–69.
46. Exacoustos C, Rosati P. Ultrasound diagnosis of uterine myomas and complications in pregnancy. Obstet Gynecol 1993;82:97–101.
47. Koetsawang S, Rachawat D, Piya-Anant M. Outcome of pregnancy in the presence of intrauterine device. Acta Obstet Gynecol Scand 1977;56:479–82.
48. Fallon JH. Pregnancy with IUD in situ. Kans Med 1985;86:322–4.
49. Mermet J, Bolcato C, Rudigoz RC, et al. Outcome of pregnancies with an intrauterine devices and their management. Rev Fr Gynecol Obstet 1986;81:233–5.
50. Abu-Yousef MM, Bleicher JJ, Williamson RA, et al. Subchorionic hemorrhage: sonographic diagnosis and clinical significance. AJR Am J Roentgenol 1987;149:737–40.
51. Bennette GL, Bromley B, Lieberman E, et al. Subchorionic hemorrhage in first-trimester pregnancies: prediction of pregnancy outcome with sonography. Radiology 1996;200:803–6.
52. Sauerbrei EE, Pham DH. Placental abruption and subchorionic hemorrhage in the first half of pregnancy: US appearance and clinical outcome. Radiology 1986;160:109–12.

53. Bloch C, Altchek A, Levy-Ravetch M. Sonography in early pregnancy: the significance of subchorionic hemorrhage. Mt Sinai J Med 1989;56:290–2.
54. Pedersen JF, Mantoni M. Prevalence and significance of subchorionic hemorrhage in threatened abortion: a sonographic study. AJR Am J Roentgenol 1990;154:535–7.
55. Maso G, D'Ottavio G, De Seta F, et al. First-trimester intrauterine hematoma and outcome of pregnancy. Obstet Gynecol 2005;105:339–44.
56. Kurtz AB, Shlansky-Goldberg RD, Choi HY, et al. Detection of retained products of conception following spontaneous abortion in the first trimester. J Ultrasound Med 1991;10:387–95.
57. Wong SF, Lam MH, Ho LC. Transvaginal sonography in the detection of retained products of conception after first-trimester spontaneous abortion. J Clin Ultrasound 2002;30:428–32.
58. Alcazar JL. Transvaginal ultrasonography combined with color velocity imaging and pulsed Doppler to detect residual trophoblastic tissue. Ultrasound Obstet Gynecol 1998;11:54–8.
59. Durfee SM, Frates MC, Luong A, et al. The sonographic and color Doppler features of retained products of conception. J Ultrasound Med 2005;24:1181–6.
60. Polat P, Suma S, Kantarcy M, et al. Color Doppler US in the evaluation of uterine vascular abnormalities. Radiographics 2002;22:47–53.
61. O'Brien P, Neyastani A, Buckley AR, et al. Uterine arteriovenous malformations: from diagnosis to treatment. J Ultrasound Med 2006;25:1387–92.
62. Huang MW, Muradali D, Thurston WA, et al. Uterine arteriovenous malformations: gray-scale and Doppler US features with MR imaging correlation. Radiology 1998;206:115–23.
63. Jain K, Fogata M. Retained products of conception mimicking a large endometrial AVM: complete resolution following spontaneous abortion. J Clin Ultrasound 2007;35:42–7.
64. Vedantham S, Goodwin SC, McLucas B, et al. Uterine artery embolization: an underused method of controlling pelvic hemorrhage. Am J Obstet Gynecol 1997;176:938–48.
65. Maleux G, Timmerman D, Heye S, et al. Acquired uterine vascular malformations: radiological and clinical outcome after transcatheter embolotherapy. Eur Radiol 2006;16:299–306.
66. Centers for Disease Control. Current trends ectopic pregnancy: United States, 1990–1992. MMWR Morb Mortal Wkly Rep 1995;44:46–8.
67. Atri M, Leduc C, Gillett P, et al. Role of endovaginal sonography in the diagnosis and management of ectopic pregnancy. Radiographics 1996;16:755–74.
68. Chavkin W. The rise in ectopic pregnancy-exploration of possible reasons. Int J Gynaecol Obstet 1982;20:341–50.
69. Bouyer J, Coste J, Shojaei T, et al. Risk factors for ectopic pregnancy: a comprehensive analysis based on a large case-control, population-based study in France. Am J Epidemiol 2003;157:185–94.
70. Urman B, Zouves C, Gomel V. Fertility outcome following tubal pregnancy. Acta Eur Fertil 1991;22:205–8.
71. Uotila J, Heinonen PK, Punnonen R. Reproductive outcome after multiple ectopic pregnancies. Int J Fertil 1989;34:102–5.
72. Gervaise A, Masson L, de Tayrac R, et al. Reproductive outcome after methotrexate treatment of tubal pregnancies. Fertil Steril 2004;82:304–8.

73. Brown DL, Doubilet PM. Transvaginal sonography for diagnosing ectopic pregnancy: positivity criteria and performance characteristics. J Ultrasound Med 1994;13:259–66.
74. Braffman BH, Coleman BG, Ramchandani P, et al. Emergency department screening for ectopic pregnancy: a prospective US study. Radiology 1994; 190:797–802.
75. Nyberg DA, Hughes MP, Mack LA, et al. Extrauterine findings of ectopic pregnancy of transvaginal US: importance of echogenic fluid. Radiology 1991;178:823–6.
76. Frates MC, Brown DL, Doubilet PM, et al. Tubal rupture in patients with ectopic pregnancy: diagnosis with transvaginal US. Radiology 1994;191:769–72.
77. Fleischer AC, Pennell RG, McKee MS, et al. Ectopic pregnancy: features at transvaginal sonography. Radiology 1990;174:375–8.
78. Frates MC, Visweswaran A, Laing FC. Comparison of tubal ring and corpus luteum echogenicities: a useful differentiating characteristic. J Ultrasound Med 2001;20:27–31.
79. Stein MW, Ricci ZJ, Novak L, et al. Sonographic comparison of the tubal ring of ectopic pregnancy with the corpus luteum. J Ultrasound Med 2004;23:57–62.
80. Atri M. Ectopic pregnancy versus corpus luteum cyst revisited: best Doppler predictors. J Ultrasound Med 2003;2:1181–4.
81. Graham M, Cooperberg PL. Ultrasound diagnosis of interstitial pregnancy: findings and pitfalls. J Clin Ultrasound 1979;7:433–7.
82. Chen GD, Lin MT, Lee MS. Diagnosis of interstitial pregnancy with sonography. J Clin Ultrasound 1994;22:439–42.
83. Kaakaji Y, Nghiem HV, Nodell C, et al. Sonography of obstetric and gynecologic emergencies: part I, obstetric emergencies. AJR Am J Roentgenol 2000;174: 641–9.
84. Ackerman TE, Levi CS, Dashefsky SM, et al. Interstitial line: sonographic finding in interstitial (cornual) ectopic pregnancy. Radiology 1993;189:83–7.
85. Jansen RP, Elliott PM. Angular intrauterine pregnancy. Obstet Gynecol 1981;58: 167–75.
86. Tarim E, Ulusan S, Kilicdag E, et al. Angular pregnancy. J Obstet Gynaecol Res 2004;30:377–9.
87. Harika G, Gabriel R, Carre-Pigeon F, et al. Primary application of three-dimensional ultrasonography to early diagnosis of ectopic pregnancy. Eur J Obstet Gynecol Reprod Biol 1995;60:117–20.
88. Izquierdo LA, Nicholas MC. Three-dimensional transvaginal sonography of interstitial pregnancy. J Clin Ultrasound 2003;31:484–7.
89. Takeuchi K, Yamada T, Oomori S, et al. Comparison of magnetic resonance imaging and ultrasonography in the early diagnosis of interstitial pregnancy. J Reprod Med 1999;44:265–8.
90. Nishino M, Hayakawa K, Kawamata K, et al. MRI of early unruptured ectopic pregnancy: detection of gestational sac. J Comput Assist Tomogr 2002;26:134–7.
91. Marcus SF, Brinsden PR. Primary ovarian pregnancy after in vitro fertilization and embryo transfer: report of seven cases. Fertil Steril 1993;60:167–9.
92. Tuncer R, Sipahi T, Erkaya S, et al. Primary twin ovarian pregnancy. Int J Gynaecol Obstet 1994;46:57–9.
93. Marret H, Hamamah S, Alonso AM, et al. Case report and review of the literature: primary twin ovarian pregnancy. Hum Reprod 1997;12:1813–5.
94. de Vries K, Shapiro I, Degani S, et al. Ovarian pregnancy in association with an intrauterine device. Int J Gynaecol Obstet 1983;21:65–70.

95. Sergent F, Mauger-Tinlot F, Gravier A, et al. Ovarian pregnancies: revaluation of diagnostic criteria. J Gynecol Obstet Biol Reprod (Paris) 2002;31:741–6.
96. Camstock C, Huston K, Lee W. The ultrasonographic appearance of ovarian ectopic pregnancies. Obstet Gynecol 2005;105:42–5.
97. Hallat JG. Primary ovarian pregnancy: a report of twenty-five cases. Am J Obstet Gynecol 1982;143:55–60.
98. Han M, Kim J, Kim H, et al. Bilateral ovarian pregnancy after in vitro fertilization and embryo transfer in a patient with tubal factor infertility. Obstet Gynecol 2005; 105:42–5.
99. Leeman LM, Wendland CL. Cervical ectopic pregnancy. Diagnosis with endovaginal ultrasound examination and successful treatment with methotrexate. Arch Fam Med 2000;9:72–7.
100. Werber J, Prasadarao PR, Harris VJ. Cervical pregnancy diagnosed by ultrasound. Radiology 1983;149:279–80.
101. Vas W, Suresh PL, Tang-Barton P, et al. Ultrasonographic differentiation of cervical abortion from cervical pregnancy. J Clin Ultrasound 1984;12:553–7.
102. Guerrier C, Wartanian R, Boblet V, et al. Cervical pregnancy. Contribution of ultrasonography to diagnosis and therapeutic management (in French). Rev Fr Gynecol Obstet 1995;90:355–9.
103. Jurkovic D, Hacket E, Campbell S. Diagnosis and treatment of early cervical pregnancy: a review and a report of two cases treated conservatively. Ultrasound Obstet Gynecol 1996;8:373–80.
104. Rafal RB, Kosovsky PA, Markisz JA. MR appearance of cervical pregnancy. J Comput Assist Tomogr 1990;14:482–4.
105. Jung SE, Byun JY, Lee JM, et al. Characteristic MR findings of cervical pregnancy. J Magn Reson Imaging 2001;13:918–22.
106. Kirk E, Bourne T. The nonsurgical management of ectopic pregnancy. Curr Opin Obstet Gynecol 2006;18:587–93.
107. Barnhart KT, Gosman G, Ashby R, et al. The medical management of ectopic pregnancy: a meta-analysis comparing "single dose" and "multidose" regimens. Obstet Gynecol 2003;101:778–84.
108. Gabbur N, Sherer DM, Hellmann M, et al. Do serum beta-human chorionic gonadotropin levels on day 4 following methotrexate treatment of patients with ectopic pregnancy predict successful single-dose therapy? Am J Perinatol 2006;23:193–6.
109. Tawfiq A, Agameya AF, Claman P. Predictors of treatment failure for ectopic pregnancy treated with single-dose methotrexate. Fertil Steril 2000;74: 877–80.
110. Menon S, Colins J, Barnhart KT. Establishing a human chorionic gonadotropin cutoff to guide methotrexate treatment of ectopic pregnancy: a systematic review. Fertil Steril 2007;87:481–4.
111. Kirk E, Condous G, Haider Z, et al. The conservative management of cervical ectopic pregnancies. Ultrasound Obstet Gynecol 2006;27:430–7.
112. Committee on Practice Bulletins-Gynecology. American College of Obstetricians and Gynaecologists. ACOG Practice Bulletin #53. Diagnosis and treatment of gestational trophoblastic disease. Obstet Gynecol 2004;103: 1365–77.
113. Soper JT, Mutch DG, Schink JC. American College of Obstetricians and Gynecologists. Diagnosis and treatment of gestational trophoblastic disease: ACOG Practice Bulletin No. 53. Gynecol Oncol 2004;93:575–85.

114. Grimes DA. Epidemiology of gestational trophoblastic disease. Am J Obstet Gynecol 1984;150:309–18.
115. Bracken MB. Incidence and aetiology of hydatidiform mole: an epidemiological review. Br J Obstet Gynaecol 1987;94:1123–35.
116. Buckley JD. The epidemiology of molar pregnancy and choriocarcinoma. Clin Obstet Gynecol 1984;27:153–9.
117. Lawler SD, Fisher RA. Genetic studies in hydatidiform mole with clinical correlations. Placenta 1987;8:77–88.
118. Lawler SD, Fisher RA, Dent J. A prospective genetic study of complete and partial hydatidiform moles. Am J Obstet Gynecol 1991;164(5 Pt 1): 1270–7.
119. Wells M. The pathology of gestational trophoblastic disease: recent advances. Pathology 2007;39:88–96.
120. Garner EI, Goldstein DP, Feltmate CM, et al. Gestational trophoblastic disease. Clin Obstet Gynecol 2007;50:112–22.
121. Wagner BJ, Woodward PJ, Dickey GE. From the archives of the AFIP. Gestational trophoblastic disease: radiologic-pathologic correlation. Radiographics 1996;16:131–48.
122. Allen SD, Lim AK, Seckl MJ, et al. Radiology of gestational trophoblastic neoplasia. Clin Radiol 2006;61:301–13.
123. Zhou Q, Lei XY, Xie Q, et al. Sonographic and Doppler imaging in the diagnosis and treatment of gestational trophoblastic disease: a 12-year experience. J Ultrasound Med 2005;24:15–24.
124. Jain KA. Gestational trophoblastic disease: pictorial review. Ultrasound Q 2005; 21:245–53.
125. Betel C, Atri M, Arenson AM, et al. Sonographic diagnosis of gestational trophoblastic disease and comparison with retained products of conception. J Ultrasound Med 2006;25:985–93.
126. Montz FJ, Schlaerth JB, Morrow CP. The natural history of theca lutein cysts. Obstet Gynecol 1988;72:247–51.
127. Ha HK, Jung JK, Jee MK, et al. Gestational trophoblastic tumors of the uterus: MR imaging-pathologic correlation. Gynecol Oncol 1995;57:340–50.

Update on Screening Breast MRI in High-Risk Women

C. Boetes, MD, PhD

KEYWORDS

• Breast • Cancer • Screening • Increased risk • MRI

Breast cancer is a major health problem in Europe and the United States. At the moment, 1 in 8 women in the Western European countries develops breast cancer during her lifetime, and approximately 30% of these women die of the disease. Although a nationwide screening program for breast cancer has shown a mortality reduction of approximately 1.2% annually in the Netherlands, mammography has a limited sensitivity especially in the dense breast, and cancers are missed at screening.[1,2]

In women with an increased risk for breast cancer, mammographic results are even more disappointing because in many cases these women are young, and younger women have often more dense breasts than postmenopausal women.

The first results regarding breast cancer screening with MRI were published by Tilanus-Linthorst and colleagues[3] in 2000. In this series, MRI detected, in 3% of the cases, a malignancy not seen on conventional imaging. After that publication, many studies were published showing the value of screening with MRI and mammography compared with screening with mammography alone in the group of women with an increased risk for breast cancer.

GENETIC COUNSELING

There are many factors that influence a woman's risk of developing breast cancer. Family history and increasing age are among the most significant risk factors. Approximately 20% to 30% of all women who have breast cancer have a relative with breast cancer.[4] Five percent to 10% of all breast cancer cases are truly hereditary.

In performing risk assessment, family history is important as is the ethnic background of a patient. For instance, women of Ashkenazi Jewish origin have an increased risk of being BRCA1 or BRCA2 carriers compared with other ethnic groups.[5]

A version of this article was previously published in *MRI Clinics* 18:2.
Department of Radiology, Maastricht University Medical Center, PO Box 5800, 6202 AZ Maastricht, the Netherlands
E-mail address: c.boetes@mumc.nl

Obstet Gynecol Clin N Am 38 (2011) 149–158
doi:10.1016/j.ogc.2011.02.007
0889-8545/11/$ – see front matter © 2011 Elsevier Inc. All rights reserved.

obgyn.theclinics.com

It is recommended that women with a likelihood of at least 10% of being a gene mutation carrier be referred for genetic counseling and testing (**Table 1**).[6,7]

There are different models used for risk assessment. The Cancer and Steroid Hormone Study is a population-based case-control study, often referred as the Claus model,[8] that fits genetic models to derive age-specific breast cancer risk assessment for women with a first-degree relative with breast cancer. The assessment of risk is based on the relative's age at diagnosis and the degree of relationship of these relatives.

Another often-used model is Gail and colleagues' model.[9] This model uses the following risk factors: age at menarche, age at first live birth, number of previous biopsies, presence of atypical hyperplasia, and number of first-degree relatives with breast cancer. There are some limitations to this model, for instance, the number of biopsies and the exclusion of more extended information about the family history. Evaluating a woman with both risk models in many cases gives discordant results.

BRCAPRO is a pedigree-based risk assessment model. BRCAPRO, however, only considers first- and second-degree family members.[10]

INDICATIONS FOR PERFORMING MRI SCREENING

Different guidelines have been published in the past decade providing indications for breast MRI in women with an increased risk for the development of breast cancer.

In the 1990s the first nonrandomized studies were initiated in the Netherlands, the United Kingdom, Canada, the United States, Italy, and Germany to determine the additional value of breast MRI to mammography in women who are BRCA1 or -2 carriers or have a lifetime risk of at least 20% to 25% for developing breast cancer. On the basis of these various retrospective studies, the American Cancer Society recommends annual MRI examination for all women with a lifetime risk of more than 20% to 25%.[11] These guidelines are completely incorporated in the guidelines of the European Society of Breast Imaging,[12] which describe in detail which groups of women should undergo breast MRI (**Box 1**).

BRCA1 AND -2 MUTATION CARRIERS

A BRCA1 mutation carrier has a lifetime risk, according the Breast Cancer Linkage Consortium (BCLC), of 87% for getting breast cancer.[13] Brose and colleagues[14]

Table 1
Criteria for referral for genetic consulting
1. One first-degree member
Breast cancer (BC) < 35   Bilateral or multicentric tumor, first tumor < 50   Ovarian cancer and BC < 70   Ovarian cancer < 50   Male BC   Breast cancer
2. Two or more relatives in the same side
Two first-degree with BC < 50   BC < 50 and ovarian cancer at any age   Prostate cancer < 60 and first-degree BC < 50   Two relatives with ovarian cancer   Three or more first-degree relatives, one < 50

Box 1
Recommendations for MRI screening together with mammography

1. BRCA mutation

2. First-degree untested relative of BRCA carrier

3. Radiation to chest wall between ages 10 and 30

4. Li-Fraumeni syndrome and first-degree relatives

5. Cowden syndrome and first-degree untested relatives

---

calculated a lower lifetime risk of approximately 73%. In the Ashkenazi Jewish women who are BRCA1 carriers, the lifetime risk is slightly lower, between 40% and 60%.[15]

In the group of BRCA1 mutation carriers, other cancers are also more frequently detected. BRCA1 carriers have a 40% to 65% cumulative risk of getting a contralateral breast cancer and a 20% to 45% risk of developing ovarian cancer.[16] Prostate cancer is probably also one of the malignancies associated with BRCA1, although less frequent than in BRCA2.[17] Male breast cancer is also seen in BRCA1 families as well as pancreatic cancer.[18] The lifetime risk for developing breast cancer in BRCA2 mutation carriers is slightly lower than in BRCA1 groups. The age at onset is slightly later.[19] According to the BCLC, the lifetime risk in BRCA2 is 84%. A large meta-analysis pooled pedigree data, however, that included more than 8000 women revealed an average cumulative breast cancer risk to age 70 in BRCA1 carriers of 65% versus 45% in BRCA2 carrier groups.[20] BRCA2 mutation carriers also have an increased risk for getting other cancers (similar to those described previously).

BRCA1-associated breast cancers are more frequently high grade and receptor status negative.[21,22] Moreover, lymphocytic infiltration is seen more often. The tumors, even when small in size, are often growing with pushing borders.[23] In contradistinction, BRCA2 breast cancer behaves more like the group of sporadic breast cancers. BRCA1 tumors often have medullary or atypical medullary features. Although *ductal carcinoma in situ* (DCIS) in and around the invasive ductal cancer is also detected in BRCA1 mutation carriers, it is less frequent than in sporadic invasive ductal cancers.[21] Unlike sporadic breast cancers where the size of the tumor is a predictor for lymph node invasion, this is not the case in BRCA1 mutation carriers.[24] Although the tumor characteristics of the BRCA1 carriers show unfavorable signs, currently there is no difference in survival between this group of women and women with a sporadic breast cancer.

SPORADIC HEREDITARY BREAST CANCER SYNDROMES

There are other, more sporadic hereditary diseases that have an increased risk for breast cancer. The Li-Fraumeni syndrome is an autosomal dominant disease causing an increased risk for developing different kinds of cancers, such as sarcoma, leukemia, and breast carcinoma. Approximately 30% of all malignancies in this syndrome develop before the age of 15, and by the age of 70 approximately 90% of the malignancies have occurred.[25,26] The Li-Fraumeni syndrome germline TP53 mutation has an unusual high prevalence in parts of Brazil. The incidence there is 1: 300 individuals.[27] Early breast cancer before age of 40 is often seen in this group of patients.

Cowden disease (multiple hamartoma syndrome) is also a rare genetic disease with an increased risk for developing breast cancer and for thyroid cancer (**Fig. 1**).[28]

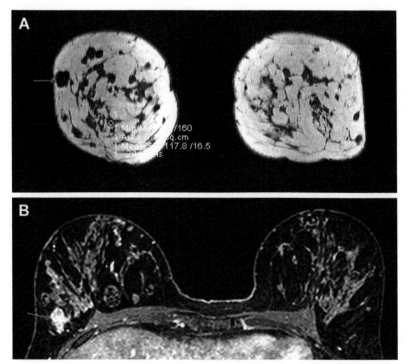

Fig. 1. (*A*) MRI performed in a patient with Cowden disease and breast cancer (*arrow*). (*B*) MRI performed in a patient with Cowden disease and breast cancer (*arrow*).

Peutz-Jeghers syndrome is characterized by hamartomatous polyps in the small bowel and also malignancies of the gastrointestinal tract and breast.[29] In Peutz-Jeghers syndrome, the lifetime risk for developing colon cancer is approximately 40%, for pancreatic cancer 35%, and for stomach cancer 30%. The risk for developing breast cancer is approximately 55%.

Muir-Torre syndrome is a variant of the hereditary nonpolyposis colon cancer. Women affected with this syndrome also have an increased risk for developing breast and endometrial cancer.

Ataxia telangiectasia is an autosomal recessive condition. Patients with this syndrome have immunodeficiency, cerebellar degeneration, and an increased risk for developing solid tumors, leukemia, and malignant lymphoma. They also have an increased risk for developing breast cancer.[30]

Patients with a family history of breast cancer tend to develop breast carcinoma at a younger age than women with no family history. The prevalence of bilateral breast cancer is also higher than seen in sporadic cases.

INDIVIDUAL INCREASED RISK

Women who received irradiation to the chest in their second or third decade of life, most for treatment of a malignant lymphoma, have a 4- to 5-fold increased risk for the development of breast cancer. In most cases, breast cancer develops approximately 20 years after the irradiation.[31] There are several other factors that increase the risk of breast cancer, such as a diagnosis of lobular carcinoma in situ (LCIS).

The lifetime risk in this group of patients may exceed 20%, but only 1 publication shows some benefit in performing breast MRI in this group of patients.[32]

In the group of patients with a diagnosis of LCIS, other risk factors, such as family history, age, and breast density, also should be considered in the decision for performing breast MRI.

A high breast density is also a risk factor for breast cancer; however, until now no data regarding the additional value of MRI in this group of women are available.

In a study published by Morris and colleagues,[33] MRI detected more mammographically occult tumors in women with a family history and a personal history for breast cancer.

Although women with a personal history of breast cancer have an increased risk, there is no sufficient evidence in support of performing MRI in this group.

TREATMENT OPTIONS

Prevention
  Prophylactic mastectomy reduces the risk for developing breast cancer by at least 90%. In this group of women, subcutaneous mastectomy is not the procedure of choice because a considerable amount of glandular tissue, especially around the nipple, is not removed. A total mastectomy is the best prevention.[34]
  Prophylactic oophorectomy reduces the risk for breast cancer in BRCA1 and BRCA2 gene carriers by approximately 50% in premenopausal women. It also reduces the risk for ovarian cancer. If prophylactic oophorectomy is performed premenopause, however, there is an increased risk for cardiovascular diseases and osteoporosis.[35]
  Chemoprevention with tamoxifen reduces the risk for breast cancer by approximately 50% but only for receptor-positive tumors.[36] The risk for receptor-negative tumors is not diminished by tamoxifen. The effect of the use of hormonal replacement therapy in BRCA1 and -2 mutation carriers is not clear.

RESULTS OF SCREENING

The first results regarding the value of screening with MRI in women with an increased risk for breast cancer were published approximately a decade ago.

Stoutjesdijk and colleagues[37] published the first results of a cohort of 179 women with a lifetime risk of 15% or more. In this series, 13 breast cancers were detected; 7 cancers were not seen on mammography, but MRI detected them all.

At the same time, Tilanus-Linthorst and colleagues[3] published the results of MRI screening in a group of 109 women with a lifetime risk of more than 25% and a breast density of more than 50%. MRI detected 3 cancers occult at mammography. In the Netherlands, approximately 20% of familial breast cancer is caused by BRCA1, 5% by BRCA2, and approximately 75% is non-BRCA1 or non-BRCA2.

The first large published study that reported on the value of MRI screening was the Dutch Magnetic Resonance Imaging Screening (MRISC) study in 2004.[38] Although the best study design would have been a randomized controlled trial with a study group of high-risk women who were screened and a control group of high-risk women who were not screened, most women will not consent to randomization. Therefore, the results from this screening study of the high-risk women were compared with a control group of nonscreened women from an external source.

This multicenter study included 1909 women: 358 women were gene carriers, 1052 women had a lifetime risk of 30% to 50% (high risk), and 499 women had a lifetime risk between 15% and 30%. Participants visited the family cancer clinic twice a year. Visit

A consisted of a clinical breast examination and visit B a clinical breast examination, mammography, and MRI.

MRI was performed in premenopausal women between days 5 and 15 of the menstrual cycle to minimize glandular tissue enhancement. Inclusion criteria included a cumulative lifetime risk of 15% or more. The women in the study were divided into 3 groups depending on their lifetime risk for breast cancer: group 1 were BRCA1 or -2 mutation carriers with an assumed lifetime risk of 60% or more; group 2 had a lifetime risk of between 30% and 50%; and group 3 had a moderate risk of between 15% and

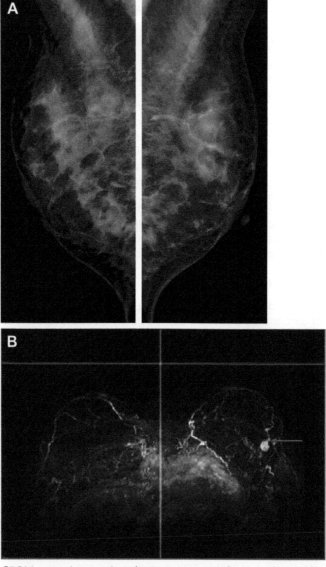

Fig. 2. (A) BRCA1 mutation carrier, dense mammography, no abnormalities. (B) MRI revealed invasive ductal carcinoma (*arrow*) in the left breast.

30%. The risk assessment was performed according the Claus tables. The age range of the women included in the study was between 25 and 70 years.

In the group of mutation carriers, 19 malignancies were detected, 16 invasive and 3 DCIS. In the high-risk group, 15 invasive malignancies were seen and no DCIS. In the moderate-risk group, 11 malignancies were found, of which 8 were invasive. In this study, the sensitivity of MRI for invasive cancer was 79.5% and of mammography was 33.3% (**Fig. 2**). The characteristics of the breast tumors detected in the study group were compared with those of 2 control groups.

The first control group was extracted from a population study investigating the frequency of BRCA mutations in a group of unselected symptomatic patients with primary breast cancer. The second group consisted of nonscreened family members with breast cancer of the participating women. The tumors in the study group were significantly smaller than in the control groups and were less likely to be node positive.

In 2005, the results of the Magnetic Resonance Imaging Breast Screening (MARIBS) trial were revealed.[39] This was also a prospective multicenter study of 649 women. Included were all gene mutation carriers and women with an annual risk of breast cancer of at least 0.9%. In this study, mammography had a sensitivity of 40% and MRI of 77%. The combined sensitivity was 94%. Therefore, annual screening with mammography and MRI detects most cancers in this group of women with a high increased risk.

At the same time, the results of a Canadian screening study were published. This study included only BRCA1 and BRCA2 mutations[40]; 236 women were included in this ultrasound investigation and 22 cancers were detected. Mammography had a sensitivity of 36%, ultrasound of 33%, and MRI of 77%. These study results also showed the superior sensitivity of MRI compared with mammography and ultrasound.

In 2007, the results from the High Breast Cancer Risk Italian Trial (HIBCRIT) were published.[41] This study included 278 women, all BRCA1 and BRCA2 carriers. Also, the sensitivity of MRI was the highest, 94% compared with the sensitivity of mammography of 59%.

Lastly, a screening study published in 2009[42] evaluated 609 high-risk women with mammography, whole breast ultrasound, and MRI. Film-screen mammography revealed a sensitivity of 33%, digital mammography 39%, and whole breast ultrasound 17%. The sensitivity of MRI was 71%. It can be concluded from this study

Table 2
Results of different screening trials

	Dutch MRISC Study, Kriege et al, 2004	Toronto, Canada, Warner et al, 2004	MARIBS	HIBCRIT Study, Sardanelli et al, 2007	Weinstein et al, 2009
CE MRI sensitivity (95% CI)	71.1% (55.7–83.6)	77.3% (54.6–92.2)	77% (60–90)	93.8% (71.7–98.9)	71.0%
XRM sensitivity	40.0% (25.7–55.7)	36.4% (17.2–59.3)	40% (24–58)	58.8% (36.0–78.4)	39.0%
CE MRI specificity	89.8% (88.9–90.7)	95.4 (93.0–97.2)	81% (80–83)		79.0%
XRM specificity	95.0% (94.3–95.6)	99.8% (98.7–100)	93% (92–95)		91.0%

Abbreviations: CE, contrast-enhanced; XRM, x-ray mammography.

that the addition of MRI to mammography in this group of patients provides the greatest potential to detect malignant tumor foci.

SUMMARY

It can be concluded that a screening MRI in asymptomatic, high-risk women plays an important role for detection of malignant tumors with an overall sensitivity of more than 70% compared with a lower sensitivity of 35% for mammography alone. The combination of mammography and MRI has the highest sensitivity (**Table 2**).

REFERENCES

1. Fracheboud J, Otto SJ, van Dijck JA, et al. Decreased rates of advanced breast cancer due to mammography screening in The Netherlands. Br J Cancer 2004; 91(5):861–7.
2. Kerlikowske K, Grady D, Barclay J, et al. Effect of age, breast density, and family history on the sensitivity of first screening mammography. JAMA 1996;276(1): 33–8.
3. Tilanus-Linthorst MM, Obdeijn IM, Bartels KC, et al. First experiences in screening women at high risk for breast cancer with MR imaging. Breast Cancer Res Treat 2000;63(1):53–60.
4. Claus EB, Schildkraut JM, Thompson WD, et al. The genetic attributable risk of breast and ovarian cancer. Cancer 1996;77(11):2318–24.
5. Struewing JP, Hartge P, Wacholder S, et al. The risk of cancer associated with specific mutations of BRCA1 and BRCA2 among Ashkenazi Jews. N Engl J Med 1997;336(20):1401–8.
6. American Society of Clinical Oncology. American Society of Clinical Oncology policy statement update: genetic testing for cancer susceptibility. J Clin Oncol 2003;21(12):2397–406.
7. Statement of the American Society of Clinical Oncology: genetic testing for cancer susceptibility, Adopted on February 20, 1996. J Clin Oncol 1996;14(5): 1730–6 [discussion: 37–40].
8. Claus EB, Risch N, Thompson WD. Autosomal dominant inheritance of early-onset breast cancer. Implications for risk prediction. Cancer 1994;73(3):643–51.
9. Gail MH, Brinton LA, Byar DP, et al. Projecting individualized probabilities of developing breast cancer for white females who are being examined annually. J Natl Cancer Inst 1989;81(24):1879–86.
10. Euhus DM, Smith KC, Robinson L, et al. Pretest prediction of BRCA1 or BRCA2 mutation by risk counselors and the computer model BRCAPRO. J Natl Cancer Inst 2002;94(11):844–51.
11. Saslow D, Boetes C, Burke W, et al. American Cancer Society guidelines for breast screening with MRI as an adjunct to mammography. CA Cancer J Clin 2007;57(2):75–89.
12. Mann RM, Kuhl CK, Kinkel K, et al. Breast MRI: guidelines from the European Society of Breast Imaging. Eur Radiol 2008;18(7):1307–18.
13. Ford D, Easton DF, Stratton M, et al. Genetic heterogeneity and penetrance analysis of the BRCA1 and BRCA2 genes in breast cancer families. The Breast Cancer Linkage Consortium. Am J Hum Genet 1998;62(3):676–89.
14. Brose MS, Rebbeck TR, Calzone KA, et al. Cancer risk estimates for BRCA1 mutation carriers identified in a risk evaluation program. J Natl Cancer Inst 2002;94(18):1365–72.

15. Warner E, Foulkes W, Goodwin P, et al. Prevalence and penetrance of BRCA1 and BRCA2 gene mutations in unselected Ashkenazi Jewish women with breast cancer. J Natl Cancer Inst 1999;91(14):1241–7.
16. Easton DF, Ford D, Bishop DT. Breast and ovarian cancer incidence in BRCA1-mutation carriers. Breast Cancer Linkage Consortium. Am J Hum Genet 1995; 56(1):265–71.
17. Edwards SM, Kote-Jarai Z, Meitz J, et al. Two percent of men with early-onset prostate cancer harbor germline mutations in the BRCA2 gene. Am J Hum Genet 2003;72(1):1–12.
18. Ozcelik H, Schmocker B, Di Nicola N, et al. Germline BRCA2 6174delT mutations in Ashkenazi Jewish pancreatic cancer patients. Nat Genet 1997;16(1):17–8.
19. Frank TS, Deffenbaugh AM, Reid JE, et al. Clinical characteristics of individuals with germline mutations in BRCA1 and BRCA2: analysis of 10,000 individuals. J Clin Oncol 2002;20(6):1480–90.
20. Antoniou A, Pharoah PD, Narod S, et al. Average risks of breast and ovarian cancer associated with BRCA1 or BRCA2 mutations detected in case Series unselected for family history: a combined analysis of 22 studies. Am J Hum Genet 2003;72(5):1117–30.
21. Pathology of familial breast cancer: differences between breast cancers in carriers of BRCA1 or BRCA2 mutations and sporadic cases. Breast Cancer Linkage Consortium. Lancet 1997;349(9064):1505–10.
22. Lakhani SR, Van De Vijver MJ, Jacquemier J, et al. The pathology of familial breast cancer: predictive value of immunohistochemical markers estrogen receptor, progesterone receptor, HER-2, and p53 in patients with mutations in BRCA1 and BRCA2. J Clin Oncol 2002;20(9):2310–8.
23. Tilanus-Linthorst M, Verhoog L, Obdeijn IM, et al. A BRCA1/2 mutation, high breast density and prominent pushing margins of a tumor independently contribute to a frequent false-negative mammography. Int J Cancer 2002; 102(1):91–5.
24. Foulkes WD, Brunet JS, Stefansson IM, et al. The prognostic implication of the basal-like (cyclin E high/p27 low/p53+/glomeruloid-microvascular-proliferation+) phenotype of BRCA1-related breast cancer. Cancer Res 2004;64(3):830–5.
25. Li FP, Fraumeni JF Jr, Mulvihill JJ, et al. A cancer family syndrome in twenty-four kindreds. Cancer Res 1988;48(18):5358–62.
26. Nichols KE, Malkin D, Garber JE, et al. Germ-line p53 mutations predispose to a wide spectrum of early-onset cancers. Cancer Epidemiol Biomarkers Prev 2001;10(2):83–7.
27. Achatz MI, Hainaut P, Ashton-Prolla P. Highly prevalent TP53 mutation predisposing to many cancers in the Brazilian population: a case for newborn screening? Lancet Oncol 2009;10(9):920–5.
28. Eng C. Genetics of Cowden syndrome: through the looking glass of oncology. Int J Oncol 1998;12(3):701–10.
29. Giardiello FM, Brensinger JD, Tersmette AC, et al. Very high risk of cancer in familial Peutz-Jeghers syndrome. Gastroenterology 2000;119(6):1447–53.
30. Athma P, Rappaport R, Swift M. Molecular genotyping shows that ataxia-telangiectasia heterozygotes are predisposed to breast cancer. Cancer Genet Cytogenet 1996;92(2):130–4.
31. Wolden SL, Hancock SL, Carlson RW, et al. Management of breast cancer after Hodgkin's disease. J Clin Oncol 2000;18(4):765–72.
32. Arpino G, Laucirica R, Elledge RM. Premalignant and in situ breast disease: biology and clinical implications. Ann Intern Med 2005;143(6):446–57.

33. Morris EA, Liberman L, Ballon DJ, et al. MRI of occult breast carcinoma in a high-risk population. AJR Am J Roentgenol 2003;181(3):619–26.
34. Hartmann LC, Sellers TA, Schaid DJ, et al. Efficacy of bilateral prophylactic mastectomy in BRCA1 and BRCA2 gene mutation carriers. J Natl Cancer Inst 2001;93(21):1633–7.
35. Kurian AW, Sigal BM, Plevritis SK. Survival analysis of cancer risk reduction strategies for BRCA1/2 mutation carriers. J Clin Oncol 2010;28(2):222–31.
36. Hemann MT, Rudolph KL, Strong MA, et al. Telomere dysfunction triggers developmentally regulated germ cell apoptosis. Mol Biol Cell 2001;12(7):2023–30.
37. Stoutjesdijk MJ, Boetes C, Jager GJ, et al. Magnetic resonance imaging and mammography in women with a hereditary risk of breast cancer. J Natl Cancer Inst 2001;93(14):1095–102.
38. Kriege M, Brekelmans CT, Boetes C, et al. Efficacy of MRI and mammography for breast-cancer screening in women with a familial or genetic predisposition. N Engl J Med 2004;351(5):427–37.
39. Leach MO, Boggis CR, Dixon AK, et al. Screening with magnetic resonance imaging and mammography of a UK population at high familial risk of breast cancer: a prospective multicentre cohort study (MARIBS). Lancet 2005; 365(9473):1769–78.
40. Warner E, Plewes DB, Hill KA, et al. Surveillance of BRCA1 and BRCA2 mutation carriers with magnetic resonance imaging, ultrasound, mammography, and clinical breast examination. JAMA 2004;292(11):1317–25.
41. Sardanelli F, Podo F, D'Agnolo G, et al. Multicenter comparative multimodality surveillance of women at genetic-familial high risk for breast cancer (HIBCRIT study): interim results. Radiology 2007;242(3):698–715.
42. Weinstein SP, Localio AR, Conant EF, et al. Multimodality screening of high-risk women: a prospective cohort study. J Clin Oncol 2009;27(36):6124–8.

Breast Magnetic Resonance Imaging: Current Clinical Indications

Eren D. Yeh, MD

KEYWORDS

• Breast • Magnetic resonance • Indications • Breast cancer

Breast cancer is the most common cancer among women. In 2009, approximately 192,370 new cases of invasive breast cancer, and an additional 62,280 in situ breast cancers, will be diagnosed. An estimated 40,170 women are expected to die from breast cancer in 2009. Because of early detection of breast cancers from widespread screening mammography and improvements in treatment, the mortality from breast cancer has decreased almost 30% since 1990.[1]

Mammography is the mainstay of breast imaging. Other imaging technologies such as ultrasound and magnetic resonance (MR) have been found to be useful adjuncts to mammography. Breast MR is highly sensitive in the detection of invasive malignancies, with reported rates of 89% to 100%, although it is somewhat limited with variable specificity, reported at 37% to 97%.[2] As technology improves, as interpretations and reporting by radiologists become standardized through the development of guidelines by expert consortiums, and as scientific investigation continues, the indications and uses of breast MR as an adjunct to mammography continue to evolve.

The specificity of breast MR has gradually improved, likely because of improved technology and increased reader experience. To standardize interpretation among radiologists and to facilitate outcome monitoring, the American College of Radiology (ACR) has developed guidelines for interpretation: the ACR BI-RADS (Breast Imaging Reporting and Data System) MR Imaging Lexicon, the first edition of the MR Imaging Lexicon, in 2003.[3] The BI-RADS MR Imaging Lexicon provides common terminology for describing findings and allows radiologists to communicate findings to referring physicians and with each other in a standardized fashion. It also facilitates comparison of findings across scientific investigations.

A version of this article was previously published in *MRI Clinics* 18:2.
Division of Breast Imaging, Department of Radiology, Brigham and Women's Hospital, Dana-Farber Cancer Institute, Harvard Medical School, 75 Francis Street, RA Building-014, Boston, MA 02115, USA
E-mail address: eyeh@partners.org

One of the current challenges that breast MR faces is that technical parameters are not standardized, varying with equipment and across practice sites, including magnet strength, pulse sequences, spatial resolution, and timing of postcontrast sequences. To address this issue, the ACR has also developed practice guidelines and technical standards for breast MR, the most recent update in 2008.[4] The ACR is also in the process of developing a breast MR accreditation program that will be part of the breast imaging accreditation program and will include technical requirements for optimal breast imaging and the requirement for an MR biopsy program. The current guidelines by the ACR are the foundation for this article on the current clinical indications for breast MR.

The ACR guidelines are designed to assist practitioners in providing appropriate radiologic care for patients.[4] They are not inflexible rules, and the ultimate judgment in determining the appropriateness of specific imaging or a specific procedure must take all circumstances into consideration. MR findings should be correlated with clinical history, physical examination, and results of mammography and other prior breast imaging.

The current guidelines published by the ACR recommend breast MR in the following circumstances[4]:

- Screening for the high-risk patient
- Screening the contralateral breast in a patient with a recently diagnosed breast malignancy
- Screening in patients with breast augmentation, for example in patients with postoperative reconstruction and previous free injections.

The diagnostic indications for breast MR are as follows:

- For extent of disease in patients with invasive carcinoma or ductal carcinoma in situ (DCIS)
- In assessing invasion deep to the fascia
- Postlumpectomy with positive margins
- Following patients with neoadjuvant chemotherapy.

In the additional evaluation of clinical or imaging findings, evaluation for recurrence of breast cancer in metastatic cancer of unknown primary or axillary adenopathy, in which a breast origin is suspected, and in lesion characterization, breast MR may be indicated when other imaging modalities, such as mammography and ultrasound, are inconclusive for the presence of breast cancer and biopsy cannot be performed. Breast MR may also be helpful for the additional evaluation of clinical or imaging findings in postoperative tissue reconstruction. Breast MR is also used for guidance for interventional procedures, such as MR core biopsy and MR-guided wire localization (**Table 1**).

SCREENING FOR THE HIGH-RISK PATIENT

In 2007, the American Cancer Society published guidelines for screening for breast cancer with MR as an adjunct to mammography.[5] The guidelines were based on several major clinical trials, the first of which was published by Kuhl and colleagues[6] in 2000, in which 192 asymptomatic women with proven or suspected BRCA mutations were enrolled in a prospective trial comparing MR with conventional imaging. Nine breast cancers were identified, 4 by mammography and ultrasound (44% sensitivity) and all 9 by MR (100% sensitivity).

Table 1
Indications for performing breast MR imaging

Breast cancer screening	Screening for the high-risk patient Contralateral breast Breast augmentation
Diagnostic indications	Extent of disease in patient with known breast cancer Following patients with neoadjuvant chemotherapy Breast cancer recurrence Metastatic cancer of unknown primary or axillary adenopathy Lesion characterization when mammography and ultrasound are inconclusive Postoperative tissue reconstruction
Procedure guidance	MR core biopsy MR-guided wire localization

Since then, there have been several studies worldwide showing benefit to screening subsets of women at high risk for breast cancer with MR.[7] In a review of 8 major clinical trials for MR screening of known or suspected BRCA 1 and BRCA 2 carriers in 4271 patients, 144 breast cancers were found with a 3% cancer yield.[8] Overall, there was a high sensitivity of MR for screening in high-risk populations, with a sensitivity of 71% to 100%, compared with 16% to 40% sensitivity with mammography. The specificity was variable. The call-back rate ranged from 8% to 17% (average 10%), with a benign biopsy rate of 3% to 15% (average 5%). **Figs. 1** and **2** show malignancies detected by screening MR in high-risk patients.

The patients at highest risk for breast cancer are those with a mutation of a breast cancer susceptibility gene. They constitute only 5% to 10% of women with breast

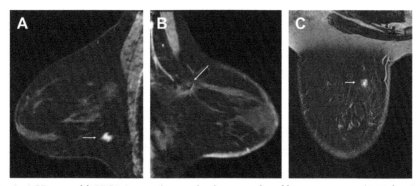

Fig. 1. A 27-year-old, BRCA 1 mutation carrier, just completed lumpectomy and XRT for right breast cancer who presented for a screening MRI. Left breast sagittal post contrast image (*A*) shows a new 0.8-cm mass with irregular margins, homogeneous enhancement and wash out kinetics. Solid mass identified on correlative ultrasound; ultrasound guided core biopsy yielded invasive ductal carcinoma. Sagittal post contrast image of the right breast (*B*) shows post treatment changes (*arrow*). Patient elected bilateral mastectomies. (*C*) A 55-year-old woman with BRCA 2 mutation who presented for a screening MR. Axial image post-contrast demonstrate a right posterior upper inner breast 1.3-cm non-mass like enhancement (*arrow*) with heterogeneous enhancement and persistent kinetics. There was no mammographic or sonographic correlate. MR core needle biopsy yielded invasive ductal carcinoma.

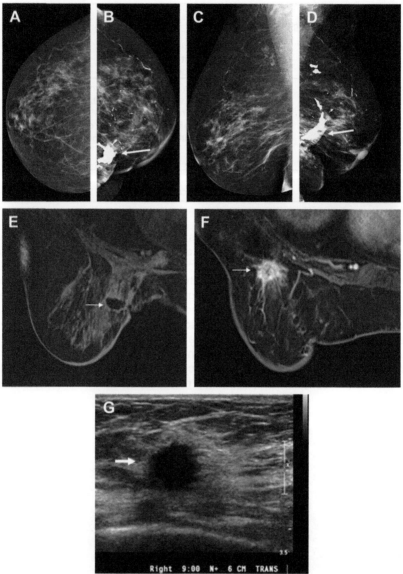

Fig. 2. A 74-year-old woman s/p right lumpectomy and XRT 31 years ago for an early stage breast cancer. Routine mammogram showed right breast post treatment changes on the cranial-caudal (CC) (*B*) and mediolateral oblique (MLO) (*D*) views, with architectural distortion and benign fat necrosis (*arrows*); the left side (*A*, CC; *C*, MLO) was negative. On MR, post treatment changes with large calcifications are present medially (*arrow*, *E*) with no enhancement at the surgical bed. A rim enhancing spiculated mass is present laterally on the post-contrast axial image (*arrow*, *F*) with rapid washout kinetics, highly suspicious for malignancy. Directed ultrasound was performed, demonstrating an 11-mm irregular solid mass in the right breast at 9:00 o'clock, which correlates with the MR finding. The mass was not seen mammographically, in retrospect, due to the far posterior location. Ultrasound core biopsy yielded invasive ductal carcinoma. The patient had a mastectomy.

cancers, but a familial genetic mutation confers a cumulative lifetime risk of breast cancer between 50% and 85% (19% risk by age 40 years, 50% risk by age 50 years, and 85% risk by age 70 years).[9] The most common of these are the BRCA 1 or 2 mutations, which account for approximately 40% to 50% of familial breast cancer; the others are caused by other familial genes that cannot be tested for at the present time.[7]

The American Cancer Society in 2007 recommended annual MR screening for breast cancer as an adjunct to mammography, based on evidence, for patients with a known BRCA mutation, patients who are a first-degree relative of a BRCA carrier, but untested, or patients with a 20% or greater lifetime risk, as defined by BRCAPRO or other models that are largely dependent on family history.[5] They recommended annual MR screening, based on expert consensus opinion, for patients with radiation to chest between the ages of 10 and 30 years, patients with Li-Fraumeni, Cowden, and Bannayan-Riley-Ruvalcaba syndromes, and first-degree relatives. They reported that there is insufficient evidence to recommend for or against MR screening in patients with a 15% to 20% lifetime risk. They also concluded that there is insufficient evidence for or against MR screening in patients with any one of these risk factors: history of lobular carcinoma in situ, atypical lobular hyperplasia, atypical ductal hyperplasia, heterogeneously or extremely dense breast tissues on mammography, and women with a personal history of breast cancer, including DCIS. They recommended against MR screening, based on expert consensus opinion, in patients with a less than 15% lifetime risk of breast cancer.

Most patients who have had radiation to the chest at a young age, between 10 and 30 years, are Hodgkin lymphoma survivors. Breast cancer is the most common second malignancy among female survivors of treated Hodgkin lymphoma, with a higher risk in those treated for Hodgkin lymphoma before age 30 years, with greater than 40 Gray dose of radiation, and with mantle field radiation compared with mediastinal radiation alone.[10,11] The risk of breast cancer approaches 29% in a woman aged 55 years who is treated for Hodgkin lymphoma at age 25 years.[10] The increased risk of secondary breast cancer emerges after a latency period of 8 to 10 years after treatment. The mammographic and sonographic appearances are similar to sporadic breast cancer; however, the malignancies tend to have unfavorable pathologic characteristics and are invasive cancers more often than DCIS. Dense breast tissues may also limit the sensitivity of screening mammography in young premenopausal women such as Hodgkin survivors. Mammography may be effective at detecting DCIS, but may be inadequate for detection of invasive breast cancer in this high-risk population. Based on expert consensus opinion, the American Cancer Society recently recommended MR imaging as an adjunct to mammography in this high-risk population.

At the Dana-Farber Cancer Institute, the authors recommend annual mammography beginning age 25 and supplement screening with MR in patients with known or suspected BRCA or familial mutations. In patients with Hodgkins lymphoma treated with mantle radiation, the authors screen beginning 8 years following treatment in patients age 25 or over and supplement screening with MR. If the patient does not live a great distance away and travel is not an impediment, the screening mammogram and MR are offset by 6 months so that the patient receives 1 screening study every 6 months, in the hope that the more frequent screening will detect a developing malignancy earlier.

Further investigation needs to be done in the subset of patients at 15% to 20% increased lifetime risk of breast cancer to determine which of these women benefit from screening MR. This group includes women with a personal history of breast cancer, including DCIS, lobular carcinoma in situ, atypical lobular hyperplasia, atypical ductal hyperplasia, and heterogeneously or extremely dense breast tissues on mammography.

SCREENING FOR THE CONTRALATERAL BREAST

Several single-institution studies have been performed in patients with a newly diagnosed invasive breast cancer with a 3% to 5% detection rate by MR of synchronous cancers in the contralateral breast (range 3%–24%), otherwise occult on clinical breast examination and mammography.[12] In a recent prospective multi-institutional trial of women with a newly diagnosed breast cancer, the American College of Radiology Imaging Network (ACRIN 6667) MRI Evaluation of the Contralateral Breast in Women Recently Diagnosed with Breast Cancer, MR detected 30 contralateral cancers among 969 women with a negative mammogram, at a rate of 3.1%.[13] The sensitivity of MR was 91%, specificity was 88%, and the negative predictive value was 99%. The biopsy rate was 12.5% (121/969), finding 30 cancers, of which 18 were invasive. The mean size of the cancers was 10.9 mm. All were small cancers with a favorable prognosis. No patients had distant metastases, and of the patients with node status known (27/30), none had positive lymph nodes. This result suggests that occult contralateral malignancies are detected by MR at an early stage that is treatable. **Fig. 3** shows a patient in whom MR detected more extensive malignancy than was originally suspected, and an occult contralateral cancer.

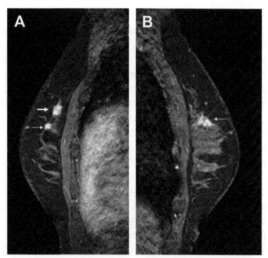

Fig. 3. A 49-year-old woman with new left breast focal asymmetry on mammography; outside ultrasound was negative. MR for problem solving demonstrates two masses in the left breast and non-mass like enhancement on the right. Sagittal post contrast image of the left breast (*A*) shows an oval 1 cm mass with irregular margins superiorly (*thick arrow*) and a second slightly inferior 0.6-cm round mass with irregular margins (*thin arrow*). MR-guided wire-localized surgical biopsies were performed: the superior mass was invasive cancer with ductal and lobular features, and the inferior mass was invasive ductal carcinoma. Sagittal image of the contralateral breast (*B*) demonstrates a mammographically occult 1.4-cm segmental non-mass like enhancement with clumped enhancement (*arrow*). MR-guided wire-localized surgical biopsy showed invasive ductal carcinoma. The patient was treated with bilateral lumpectomies and XRT. (*From* Raza S, Birdwell RL, Ritner JA, et al. Specialty imaging: breast MR: a comprehensive imaging guide. Salt Lake City, UT: Amirsys; 2010. p. 98; with permission.)

If a contralateral suspicious lesion is detected at MR, it is essential that biopsy diagnosis be established before surgical planning, as not all suspicious lesions are malignant.

IMPLANTS AND BREAST AUGMENTATION

Screening MR may be helpful in patients with augmentation or cosmetic injections. MR has been shown to better visualize tissue around a silicone implant.[14] Detection of malignancy may be challenging with mammography in patients with free injection of materials such as silicone, paraffin, or polyacrylamide gel; MR in these cases may detect malignancy to better advantage. MR may also detect malignancies that occur posterior to an implant, which would not be visualized mammographically because of the posterior location.

MR imaging has been shown to have the highest sensitivity and specificity for the diagnosis of silicone implant rupture without the use ionizing radiation. Sensitivity ranges from 28% to 59% for mammography, and 78% to 81% for MR.[15,16] To optimize detection of implant rupture, no contrast is given to the patient- and silicone-selective sequences, and water-suppression techniques are used. If the clinical indication is to evaluate for possible implant rupture, the technique is not designed to evaluate for breast cancer, as no contrast is given to the patient and the sequences are not optimized for breast cancer detection.

When an implant is surgically placed, the body forms a fibrous capsule of scar tissue around the implant. In patients with a saline implant, a rupture will be clinically evident, with a decrease in the size and contour of the breast, and no imaging will be necessary. In patients with a silicone implant, the implant may be intact, or there may be an intracapsular or an extracapsular rupture. Most silicone implants more than 10 years old have a rupture, most commonly intracapsular. An intracapsular rupture occurs when the envelope breaks, but the silicone remains contained by the fibrous capsule. This may be seen as a linguine sign on MR imaging. Signs of an incomplete envelope collapse on MR are the subcapsular line sign, teardrop sign, and keyhole sign.[17]

An extracapsular rupture represents extrusion of silicone outside the fibrous capsule. On breast MR, silicone may be seen within the breast tissues outside the implant or in the axillary lymph nodes. The signal intensities on the MR sequences obtained will follow silicone.

EXTENT OF DISEASE

MR has been shown in several studies to be more sensitive than physical examination and conventional imaging, including mammography and ultrasound, in determining the extent of disease in patients newly diagnosed with breast cancer. It has been found to be more accurate than mammography, ultrasound, and clinical examination in assessing primary tumor size. MR depicts otherwise unsuspected sites of cancer in 16% (range 6%–34%).[12] **Figs. 3** and **4** show patients in whom MR detected more extensive disease than was originally suspected by conventional imaging.

A recent meta-analysis, including 19 published studies of 2610 women with newly diagnosed breast cancer undergoing preoperative MR, detected multifocal or multicentric cancer occult to conventional imaging in 16% of the patients.[18] MR had a high specificity in this analysis, with 66% of suspicious MR lesions pathologically proven to be malignant. In patients who are possible lumpectomy candidates, determining the extent of disease is important in surgical planning, as the goal is to completely excise the tumor with clean margins with as few surgical procedures as

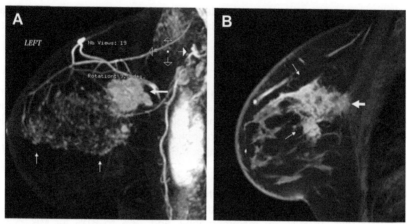

Fig. 4. Two different patients demonstrating extent of disease on MR. (*A*) A 33-year-old woman who presented with a lump and 3.3-cm mass by mammogram and ultrasound. MR shows the known mass (*large arrow*) with adjacent extensive regional clumped non-mass like enhancement extending to the nipple (*small arrow*), best seen on the MIP image (*A*). Ultrasound core biopsy yielded invasive ductal carcinoma. The patient was treated with neoadjuvant chemotherapy. (*B*) A 46-year-old woman with a lump. On the sagittal post contrast image, there is a large enhancing mass with spiculated margins and wash out kinetics (*thin arrows*). There is tenting and enhancement of the adjacent pectoralis muscle, suggesting invasion of the muscle (*thick arrow*). Ultrasound guided core biopsy yielded invasive ductal carcinoma. The patient underwent a mastectomy and invasion of pectoralis muscle with tumor was found.

possible. MR has been beneficial in improving surgical planning when assessing for extent of disease.

Patient treatment has been reported to have changed after preoperative MR in 11% to 28% of patients, usually conversion from planned breast conservation to mastectomy.[19,20] In the meta-analysis by Houssami and colleagues,[18] a subset of 13 studies assessed the effect of MR staging on surgical treatment. They found that 11.3% of women were converted from lumpectomy to more extensive surgery, wider or additional excision, or mastectomy, and 8.1% of the women were converted from lumpectomy to mastectomy because of additional sites of malignancy detected with MR.

In posterior breast cancers, assessment of pectoralis muscle invasion is important for surgical planning. MR is the most accurate imaging method for assessing the chest wall and for pectoralis muscle involvement, with a 71% to 100% positive predictive value for pectoralis muscle involvement.[21,22] In patients with posterior breast tumors, signs suggestive of pectoralis muscle invasion are obliteration of the fat plane between the tumor and muscle, and abnormal enhancement of the pectoralis muscle. **Fig. 4**B shows a patient with pectoralis muscle invasion.

MR has been found to be helpful in assessing the extent of disease in cases of invasive lobular carcinoma, in patients with dense breast tissues, and in patients with extensive intraductal component (EIC). Invasive lobular carcinoma histologically has tumor cells infiltrating the stroma in a single-file fashion, and can often be occult to physical examination, mammography, ultrasound, and MR because of its insidious pattern of infiltration.[23,24] MR has been found to be significantly more accurate than mammography (85% compared with 32%) in assessing size and extent of tumor in invasive lobular carcinoma.[25] A recently published study reviewed the current literature on invasive lobular carcinoma to assess the usefulness of MR in the workup of invasive lobular carcinoma, performing a meta-analysis when possible.[26] They found additional ipsilateral lesions detected in 32% of patients and 7% contralateral lesions occult to other modalities, with a sensitivity of 93% and a correlation with pathology ranging from 0.81 to 0.97. The MR findings changed surgical management in 28% of the cases. MR therefore may be helpful in preoperative planning of invasive lobular carcinoma, particularly when breast conservation is being considered.

Young patients and patients with dense breast tissues mammographically and a newly diagnosed cancer may benefit from preoperative MR. MR has been found to be more accurate than mammography in assessing tumor extent in patients with dense breast tissues. In one study of patients with multifocal or multicentric carcinoma and dense breast tissues, mammography detected the additional sites of malignancy in 35% and MR 100%.[27]

Invasive breast carcinomas with EIC are associated with DCIS-involved surgical margins and have an increased recurrence rate. The EIC component is nonpalpable, and the size is frequently underestimated on mammography. MR has been found to be more accurate in assessing extent of disease in invasive breast cancers with EIC.[28–30]

Preoperative breast MR to assess extent of disease is particularly important in those patients in whom breast conservation with partial breast irradiation is a treatment consideration. In an effort to decrease the side effects of conventional whole-breast irradiation in lumpectomy patients, investigations are currently ongoing with partial breast irradiation. In a study of 79 patients with breast cancer who were potential candidates for lumpectomy and accelerated partial breast irradiation, additional sites of cancer were observed in 30 patients (38%) on preoperative MR, occult to physical examination and mammography.[31] Of these, 8 (10%) had a malignancy in a different quadrant than the index tumor. The additional sites of occult malignancy would have been outside the treatment area covered by the partial breast irradiation.

To date, there have not been any randomized prospective trials published in the literature assessing the effect of breast MR on mastectomy rates or long-term outcomes such as recurrence rates or mortality. Several studies have shown that additional sites of disease can be found with preoperative MR. However, at this time, it is not certain in which subsets of patients the addition of preoperative MR imaging will result in improved overall survival.

There have been 2 retrospective studies assessing the effect of preoperative breast MR on long-term outcomes. In a study comparing 346 patients, 121 patients of whom had a preoperative MR and 225 patients who did not have a preoperative MR, the in-breast tumor recurrence rate was significantly lower; 1.2% in the patients with the preoperative MR compared with 6.8% in patients without the preoperative MR.[32] The investigators concluded that preoperative MR of the breast is recommended in patients with histopathologically verified breast cancer for local staging. A limitation of the study was that the data were not adjusted for tumor size, nodal status, or use of systemic therapy between groups.

In a more recently published work, 756 women with early-stage invasive breast carcinoma or DCIS who underwent breast-conserving therapy with definitive breast irradiation were studied.[33] Of these, 215 had preoperative breast MR, and 541 women did not. No difference was found in the 8-year local failure rate (3% vs 4%), no difference in overall survival (86% vs 87%), and no difference in freedom from metastases (89% vs 92%). Their conclusion was that preoperative breast MR was not associated with an improvement in outcome after breast conservation with radiation. Limitations of the study were that it was nonrandomized and retrospective. In addition, patients with extensive disease on MR imaging who underwent mastectomy were excluded from the study, which may underestimate the value of MR.

When additional findings are identified at MR, it is important to have a biopsy diagnosis before surgical planning. False-positive enhancing lesions may be the result of benign lesions such as fibroadenomas, sclerosing adenosis, fat necrosis, fibrocystic changes, and normal breast tissue. Multidisciplinary discussions including the surgeon, medical oncologist, radiation oncologist, radiologist, and pathologist are important in the optimal care of patients, and in decisions regarding additional MR imaging findings before changing management, to avoid unnecessary wider excisions or mastectomy.

FOLLOWING NEOADJUVANT CHEMOTHERAPY

Several studies have shown that MR is more accurate than physical examination, mammography, and ultrasound in monitoring response to neoadjuvant chemotherapy in patients with large breast cancers. Survival has been shown to be equivalent in patients with palpable breast cancers undergoing conventional chemotherapy after treatment and those undergoing chemotherapy before surgery, also known as neoadjuvant chemotherapy, followed by surgery and radiation.[34,35]

Potential advantages to having chemotherapy before surgery are reduction of tumor volume permitting breast conservation surgery, earlier treatment of micrometastatic disease, and assessment of tumor response in vivo to specific chemotherapeutic regimens, which may permit the oncologist to tailor preoperative or postoperative chemotherapy more effectively. If the tumor responds early to treatment, then it can be continued, whereas if the tumor does not respond, then the toxic therapy can be changed earlier in the course of treatment. It also allows for the study of biologic markers that may predict response.

MR is helpful when diagnosing a new malignancy before treatment. It can determine size and location of primary tumor, extent of disease, possible nodal involvement, chest wall invasion, and evaluate the contralateral breast for occult disease.

MR during or at the conclusion of chemotherapeutic treatment before surgery is helpful when performed to assess response. MR can distinguish responders from nonresponders. Decrease in tumor size and decrease in tumor vascularity suggest response.

If the tumor is not responding to specific chemotherapeutic agents, changes can be made earlier in the course of treatment so the patient does not continue to receive toxic therapy that is ineffective in reducing the tumor burden. After treatment, the breast MR tumor size correlation with pathology at surgery has been shown to be $r = 0.75$ to 0.93; more accurate than physical examination, mammography, and ultrasound.[36–39] Accurate prediction of residual tumor size following neoadjuvant chemotherapy is helpful in surgical planning. Among other things, the surgeons need to determine whether the patient is a candidate for lumpectomy and radiation therapy versus mastectomy, and to determine the amount of tissue that needs to be excised during surgery to attain clean margins. **Fig. 5** shows a patient who received neoadjuvant chemotherapy.

MR is not perfect and can overestimate or underestimate residual disease.[36] In cases in which MR overestimates residual disease, the residual enhancement may be caused by reactive inflammation and tumor response and healing. Chemotherapy-induced fibrosis can be difficult to differentiate from residual disease.[40] In cases in which MR underestimates residual disease, decreased enhancement may be the result of small foci of invasive cancer, nests of tumor, or

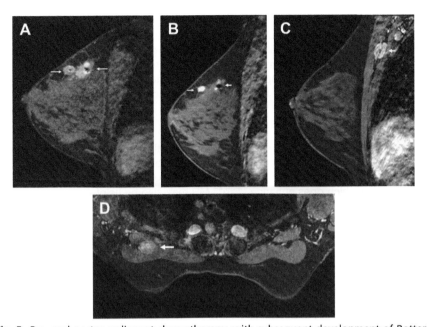

Fig. 5. Pre- and postneoadjuvant chemotherapy, with subsequent development of Rotter's node. A 31-year-old woman presented with a lump. Ultrasound guided core biopsy of two adjacent masses demonstrated invasive ductal carcinoma, poorly differentiated. Sagittal post contrast MR image (*A*) performed prior to neoadjuvant chemotherapy demonstrated the known malignancy, measuring 3.8-cm by MR with artifact from two clips from prior ultrasound guided core biopsies. Following neoadjuvant chemotherapy, a 1-cm residual enhancing mass is present anteriorly on the post contrast sagittal MR (*B, thin arrow*) with artifact from clip posteriorly and minimal posterior enhancement (*B, thick arrow*). The patient was treated with lumpectomy and XRT. She was asymptomatic for two years. On follow up MR a new 2 cm Rotter's node, between the pectoralis major and minor muscles (*C*, sagittal post contrast image; *D*, axial delayed post contrast image) was seen. She subsequently had a left axillary lymph node dissection with 1/14 lymph nodes positives (the Rotter's node was positive).

subtypes such as lobular carcinoma, which have been shown to have variable enhancement on MR.[23,41,42] Gadolinium uptake is related to tumor angiogenesis and neovascularity, and lack of these in DCIS may explain the variable uptake seen in residual DCIS.

Certain chemotherapeutic agents may affect the tumor physiology by changing tumor vascularization and vascular permeability, thereby changing MR imaging characteristics. One study has suggested that residual disease on MR is frequently underestimated in tumors treated with taxane-containing regimens.[43] Tumor physiology can potentially be used to optimize the sequence of neoadjuvant chemotherapy in breast cancer. It has been hypothesized that tumors with high interstitial fluid pressure or hypoxia respond poorly to chemotherapy because of poor drug delivery. Paclitaxel significantly reduced the interstitial fluid pressure and improved the oxygenation of tumors, whereas doxorubicin did not cause any significant change.[44]

Clip placement within the tumor mass is crucial before treatment with neoadjuvant chemotherapy, as the tumor may have a complete radiologic and pathologic response. Surgical excision is performed unless the patient has known metastatic cancer, to assess pathologically the extent of residual tumor and to remove all known malignancy. If the tumor is not visible by imaging following neoadjuvant chemotherapy, the clip is used to guide wire-localized surgical excision. The pathologist also uses the clip as a guide in locating the original tumor bed to assess response. Tumor response to chemotherapy is a predictor of outcome and complete pathologic responders have a significantly better long-term outcome.

EVALUATION FOR RECURRENCE OF BREAST CANCER

Several studies have shown benefits of MR in differentiating scar versus recurrence at the umpectomy site in patients in whom mammography is indeterminate. Scar older than 6 months postoperatively tends not to enhance with gadolinium, as opposed to malignancy which does enhance.[14,45,46] MR may also be helpful when recurrence is suspected in the setting of postoperative tissue reconstruction with an autologous flap or a silicone implant reconstruction. **Fig. 6** shows a patient *status/post* (s/p) mastectomy and implant reconstruction with a recurrence detected by MR.

METASTATIC CANCER OF UNKNOWN PRIMARY AND AXILLARY ADENOPATHY

The incidence of axillary metastases from an occult primary breast cancer is low; less than 1% of breast cancers.[47] In the past, mastectomy with axillary node dissection or, less commonly, whole breast radiation were the most common treatments in patients with axillary nodal metastases from an adenocarcinoma with an unknown primary site. However, in approximately one-third of cases, no tumor is found at pathologic evaluation of the mastectomy specimen.[48–50]

Breast MR has been shown to identify a primary breast tumor in 70% to 86% of clinically, mammographically, and ultrasound occult primary breast tumors in patients

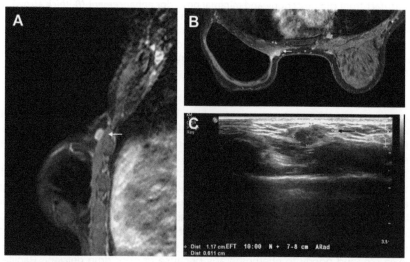

Fig. 6. A 44-year-old asymptomatic woman s/p left mastectomy and saline implant, recently finished treatment. Postcontrast MR shows the mastectomy with saline implant and 1-cm oval enhancing mass in the left superior medial breast (*A*, sagittal; *B*, axial). Focal ultrasound of the MR finding showed a 1-cm solid mass with irregular margins (*C*). Fine-needle aspiration (FNA) was performed with cytology positive for malignancy, consistent with a recurrence.

presenting with metastatic adenopathy of unknown primary.[51–53] The tumor size tends to be small, less than 2 cm. Clinical treatment decisions can be altered by results from the breast MR. If a breast primary malignancy is found, breast conservation may be a treatment option.[54] If the breast MR is negative, mastectomy may not be necessary as a negative breast MR is predictive of a low tumor yield at mastectomy.[50]

Chemotherapeutic regimens would also be tailored to breast cancer if a primary breast malignancy is identified. Moreover, these are often less toxic than chemotherapeutic regimens for an adenocarcinoma of unknown primary. Patients with breast cancer tend to have a more favorable prognosis than other adenocarcinomas; prognostic information is helpful to clinicians in counseling patients.

MR is therefore helpful in determining the presence of an occult primary breast cancer when there are malignant adenocarcinoma axillary metastases and negative physical examination and mammogram. **Fig. 7** shows a patient with malignant axillary adenopathy and occult primary malignancy detected by MR.

PROBLEM SOLVING

MR has been shown to be helpful as a problem-solving tool in cases in which the mammographic and sonographic findings are inconclusive despite a thorough diagnostic workup.[55,56] For example, MR may be performed for problem solving if an asymmetry is seen on 1 view only and cannot be three-dimensionally localized for a mammographic- or sonographic-guided biopsy. In a recent retrospective review of MR examinations with the indication of problem solving for inconclusive findings on mammography, the equivocal findings most frequently leading to MR were asymmetry and architectural distortion.[57] No suspicious MR correlate was found in 100 of 115 cases (87%). In cases in which the breast MR is negative, a final reported recommendation to the referring clinician must be made for the patient's imaging studies.

In the study discussed earlier, MR identified 15 enhancing masses (13%) that correlated with the mammographic abnormality; of these, 6 were malignant.[57] Eighteen (15.7%) incidental lesions were found, all of which were benign. The investigators concluded that breast MR is a useful adjunct when conventional imaging is equivocal,

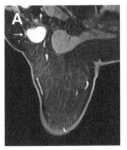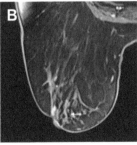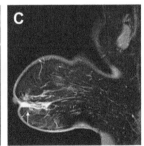

Fig. 7. A 76-year-old woman with prior right mastectomy 20 years ago, presents with new left axillary lymphadenopathy. Ultrasound core biopsy of the lymph node yielded metastatic lobular carcinoma, consistent with spread from a breast carcinoma. MR was performed to assess for breast primary, occult to physical examination and mammogram. MR showed enlarged left axillary lymph node (A) with retroareolar 1.0-cm linear enhancement, on the post contrast axial (B) and sagittal (C) images with persistent delayed kinetics. MR core biopsy yielded invasive lobular carcinoma. Patient had a left modified radical mastectomy with axillary dissection. Pathology was invasive lobular carcinoma, 1.6-cm and 1/14 lymph nodes positive.

but caution that strict patient selection criteria are necessary because of the high frequency of false positives. **Fig. 8** shows a patient in whom MR was helpful in problem solving.

MR may also be helpful postoperatively, when additional tumor is suspected to be present within the breast, such as in cases of positive margins or normal breast tissue at pathology. MR is helpful for surgical planning when additional surgery is expected. **Fig. 9** shows a patient in whom malignancy was suspected and an MR was helpful for surgical planning before re-excision.

MR PROCEDURE GUIDANCE

When lesions are identified on breast MR that are occult on mammography and ultrasound, MR is indicated for guidance of interventional procedures such as MR-guided

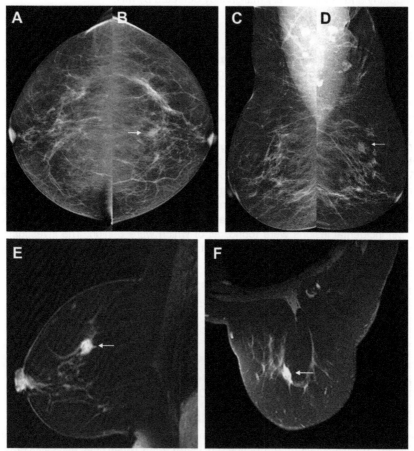

Fig. 8. A 83-year-old woman with right breast focal asymmetry (*arrow*) on mammogram (*B*, right CC; *D*, right MLO, arrows. Left CC (*A*); and MLO (*C*) views are normal) for which MR imaging was recommended. Ultrasound was negative. On MR, a mass with spiculated margins and internal enhancing septations was noted on the sagittal postcontrast. (*E*) and axial delayed postcontrast (*F*) images, wash-out kinetics. Stereotactic core biopsy was performed on the mammographic finding, with pathology of invasive lobular carcinoma. The patient elected mastectomy.

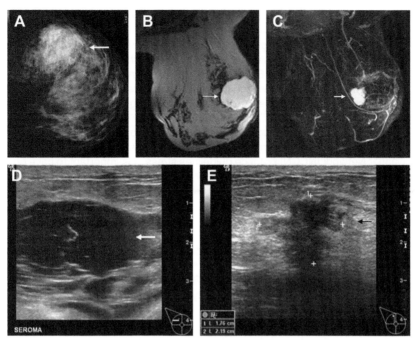

Fig. 9. A 58-year-old woman with recently diagnosed right breast cancer s/p right breast surgical excision at outside hospital with normal breast tissue at pathology, who presented for imaging evaluation to assess for residual tumor. CC view on mammogram (*A*) shows dense breast tissues with a mass laterally (*arrow*). Ultrasound (not shown) showed a seroma. Axial T2-weighted MR image with fat suppression shows a seroma laterally (*B*, *arrow*). Post-contrast axial MIP image shows an enhancing mass at the medial aspect of the seroma cavity. Focal ultrasound was subsequently performed, showing the seroma (*D*) with 2.2-cm irregular hypoechoic mass at the medial aspect of the cavity (*E*). Ultrasound-guided wire-localized surgical excision was performed with confirmation of removal of the malignancy at pathology.

percutaneous core biopsy and MR-guided preoperative wire localization for surgical excision. MR procedures may also be performed in cases in which the MR finding is more confidently seen on MR than on other imaging modalities. It is important to have MR biopsy capability for lesions detected only on MR; this will be a requirement in the new ACR breast MR accreditation program.

SUMMARY

Indications for breast MR continue to evolve as technology improves, interpretations become more standardized, and scientific investigation continues. MR should not be used in place of a full mammographic and sonographic workup. MR is useful as an adjunct to mammography in high-risk screening patients with a lifetime risk greater than 20% to 25%, including BRCA 1 and 2 patients, Hodgkin survivors treated with mantle radiation, patients with unknown primary and axillary metastases, problem solving, and in following response to treatment in patients receiving neoadjuvant chemotherapy. It is currently unclear in which subset of patients with a previous personal history of breast cancer screening is beneficial, or whether patients with intermediate risk factors, such as a previous biopsy diagnosis of atypical lobular hyperplasia or lobular carcinoma in situ, should be screened.

Not all patients with newly diagnosed breast cancer should undergo MR. The potential false positives must be considered and discussed with the patient before recommending MR. The Comparative Effectiveness of MRI in Breast Cancer (COMICE) trial in the United Kingdom is a randomized trial of 1850 patients in progress to evaluate the effect of MR on selection of patients for breast-conserving therapy and the adequacy of breast-conservation surgery.[19]

Further randomized, prospective clinical trials need to be performed to address questions and further delineate indications for breast MR. As the National Comprehensive Cancer Network (NCCN) practice guidelines stress, it is important to have proper equipment, imaging technique, and provider training to achieve high-quality breast MR.[58]

REFERENCES

1. American Cancer Society. 2009. Available at: http://www.cancer.org. Accessed 2009.
2. Kuhl C. The current status of breast MR imaging. Part I. Choice of technique, image interpretation, diagnostic accuracy, and transfer to clinical practice. Radiology 2007;244(2):356–78.
3. American College of Radiology. ACR Breast Imaging Reporting and Data System (BIRADS): breast imaging atlas. 4th edition. Reston (VA): American College of Radiology; 2003.
4. American College of Radiology. Available at: http://www.acr.org. Accessed 2009.
5. Saslow D, Boetes C, Burke W, et al. American Cancer Society guidelines for breast screening with MRI as an adjunct to mammography. CA Cancer J Clin 2007;57(2):75–89.
6. Kuhl CK, Schmutzler RK, Leutner CC, et al. Breast MR imaging screening in 192 women proved or suspected to be carriers of a breast cancer susceptibility gene: preliminary results. Radiology 2000;215(1):267–79.
7. Kuhl CK. Current status of breast MR imaging. Part 2. Clinical applications. Radiology 2007;244(3):672–91.
8. Lehman CD. Role of MRI in screening women at high risk for breast cancer. J Magn Reson Imaging 2006;24(5):964–70.
9. Liberman L. Breast cancer screening with MRI—what are the data for patients at high risk? N Engl J Med 2004;351(5):497–500.
10. Lee L, Pintilie M, Hodgson DC, et al. Screening mammography for young women treated with supradiaphragmatic radiation for Hodgkin's lymphoma. Ann Oncol 2008;19(1):62–7.
11. De Bruin ML, Sparidans J, van't Veer MB, et al. Breast cancer risk in female survivors of Hodgkin's lymphoma: lower risk after smaller radiation volumes. J Clin Oncol 2009;27(26):4239–46.
12. Liberman L. Breast MR imaging in assessing extent of disease. Magn Reson Imaging Clin N Am 2006;14(3):339–49, vi.
13. Lehman CD, Gatsonis C, Kuhl CK, et al. MRI evaluation of the contralateral breast in women with recently diagnosed breast cancer. N Engl J Med 2007;356(13): 1295–303.
14. Heywang SH, Hilbertz T, Beck R, et al. Gd-DTPA enhanced MR imaging of the breast in patients with postoperative scarring and silicon implants. J Comput Assist Tomogr 1990;14(3):348–56.

15. Goodman CM, Cohen V, Thornby J, et al. The life span of silicone gel breast implants and a comparison of mammography, ultrasonography, and magnetic resonance imaging in detecting implant rupture: a meta-analysis. Ann Plast Surg 1998;41(6):577–85 [discussion: 585–576].

16. Ikeda DM, Borofsky HB, Herfkens RJ, et al. Silicone breast implant rupture: pitfalls of magnetic resonance imaging and relative efficacies of magnetic resonance, mammography, and ultrasound. Plast Reconstr Surg 1999;104(7): 2054–62.

17. Soo MS, Kornguth PJ, Walsh R, et al. Intracapsular implant rupture: MR findings of incomplete shell collapse. J Magn Reson Imaging 1997;7(4):724–30.

18. Houssami N, Ciatto S, Macaskill P, et al. Accuracy and surgical impact of magnetic resonance imaging in breast cancer staging: systematic review and meta-analysis in detection of multifocal and multicentric cancer. J Clin Oncol 2008;26(19):3248–58.

19. Orel S. Who should have breast magnetic resonance imaging evaluation? J Clin Oncol 2008;26(5):703–11.

20. Braun M, Polcher M, Schrading S, et al. Influence of preoperative MRI on the surgical management of patients with operable breast cancer. Breast Cancer Res Treat 2008;111(1):179–87.

21. Morris EA, Schwartz LH, Drotman MB, et al. Evaluation of pectoralis major muscle in patients with posterior breast tumors on breast MR images: early experience. Radiology 2000;214(1):67–72.

22. Kazama T, Nakamura S, Doi O, et al. Prospective evaluation of pectoralis muscle invasion of breast cancer by MR imaging. Breast Cancer 2005;12(4):312–6.

23. Yeh ED, Slanetz PJ, Edmister WB, et al. Invasive lobular carcinoma: spectrum of enhancement and morphology on magnetic resonance imaging. Breast J 2003; 9(1):13–8.

24. Kumar V, Abbas AK, Fausto N, et al. Robbins and Cotran pathologic basis of disease. 7th edition. Philadelphia: Elsevier Saunders; 2005.

25. Rodenko GN, Harms SE, Pruneda JM, et al. MR imaging in the management before surgery of lobular carcinoma of the breast: correlation with pathology. AJR Am J Roentgenol 1996;167(6):1415–9.

26. Mann RM, Hoogeveen YL, Blickman JG, et al. MRI compared to conventional diagnostic work-up in the detection and evaluation of invasive lobular carcinoma of the breast: a review of existing literature. Breast Cancer Res Treat 2008;107(1): 1–14.

27. Van Goethem M, Schelfout K, Dijckmans L, et al. MR mammography in the preoperative staging of breast cancer in patients with dense breast tissue: comparison with mammography and ultrasound. Eur Radiol 2004;14(5):809–16.

28. Ikeda O, Nishimura R, Miyayama H, et al. Magnetic resonance evaluation of the presence of an extensive intraductal component in breast cancer. Acta Radiol 2004;45(7):721–5.

29. Van Goethem M, Schelfout K, Kersschot E, et al. MR mammography is useful in the preoperative locoregional staging of breast carcinomas with extensive intraductal component. Eur J Radiol 2007;62(2):273–82.

30. Schouten van der Velden AP, Boetes C, Bult P, et al. Magnetic resonance imaging in size assessment of invasive breast carcinoma with an extensive intraductal component. BMC Med Imaging 2009;9:5.

31. Godinez J, Gombos EC, Chikarmane SA, et al. Breast MRI in the evaluation of eligibility for accelerated partial breast irradiation. AJR Am J Roentgenol 2008; 191(1):272–7.

32. Fischer U, Zachariae O, Baum F, et al. The influence of preoperative MRI of the breasts on recurrence rate in patients with breast cancer. Eur Radiol 2004; 14(10):1725–31.

33. Solin LJ, Orel SG, Hwang WT, et al. Relationship of breast magnetic resonance imaging to outcome after breast-conservation treatment with radiation for women with early-stage invasive breast carcinoma or ductal carcinoma in situ. J Clin Oncol 2008;26(3):386–91.

34. Fisher B, Bryant J, Wolmark N, et al. Effect of preoperative chemotherapy on the outcome of women with operable breast cancer. J Clin Oncol 1998;16(8): 2672–85.

35. Bonadonna G, Valagussa P. Primary chemotherapy in operable breast cancer. Semin Oncol 1996;23(4):464–74.

36. Yeh E, Slanetz P, Kopans DB, et al. Prospective comparison of mammography, sonography, and MRI in patients undergoing neoadjuvant chemotherapy for palpable breast cancer. AJR Am J Roentgenol 2005;184(3): 868–77.

37. Segara D, Krop IE, Garber JE, et al. Does MRI predict pathologic tumor response in women with breast cancer undergoing preoperative chemotherapy? J Surg Oncol 2007;96(6):474–80.

38. Rosen EL, Blackwell KL, Baker JA, et al. Accuracy of MRI in the detection of residual breast cancer after neoadjuvant chemotherapy. AJR Am J Roentgenol 2003;181(5):1275–82.

39. Partridge SC, Gibbs JE, Lu Y, et al. Accuracy of MR imaging for revealing residual breast cancer in patients who have undergone neoadjuvant chemotherapy. AJR Am J Roentgenol 2002;179(5):1193–9.

40. Helvie MA, Joynt LK, Cody RL, et al. Locally advanced breast carcinoma: accuracy of mammography versus clinical examination in the prediction of residual disease after chemotherapy. Radiology 1996;198(2):327–32.

41. Qayyum A, Birdwell RL, Daniel BL, et al. MR imaging features of infiltrating lobular carcinoma of the breast: histopathologic correlation. AJR Am J Roentgenol 2002; 178(5):1227–32.

42. Weinstein SP, Orel SG, Heller R, et al. MR imaging of the breast in patients with invasive lobular carcinoma. AJR Am J Roentgenol 2001;176(2):399–406.

43. Denis F, Desbiez-Bourcier AV, Chapiron C, et al. Contrast enhanced magnetic resonance imaging underestimates residual disease following neoadjuvant docetaxel based chemotherapy for breast cancer. Eur J Surg Oncol 2004;30(10): 1069–76.

44. Taghian AG, Abi-Raad R, Assaad SI, et al. Paclitaxel decreases the interstitial fluid pressure and improves oxygenation in breast cancers in patients treated with neoadjuvant chemotherapy: clinical implications. J Clin Oncol 2005;23(9): 1951–61.

45. Gilles R, Guinebretiere JM, Shapeero LG, et al. Assessment of breast cancer recurrence with contrast-enhanced subtraction MR imaging: preliminary results in 26 patients. Radiology 1993;188(2):473–8.

46. Dao TH, Rahmouni A, Campana F, et al. Tumor recurrence versus fibrosis in the irradiated breast: differentiation with dynamic gadolinium-enhanced MR imaging. Radiology 1993;187(3):751–5.

47. Harris JR. Diseases of the breast. 3rd edition. Philadelphia: Lippincott Williams & Wilkins; 2004.

48. Jackson B, Scott-Conner C, Moulder J. Axillary metastasis from occult breast carcinoma: diagnosis and management. Am Surg 1995;61(5):431–4.

49. Fortunato L, Sorrento JJ, Golub RA, et al. Occult breast cancer. A case report and review of the literature. N Y State J Med 1992;92(12):555–7.
50. Olson JA Jr, Morris EA, Van Zee KJ, et al. Magnetic resonance imaging facilitates breast conservation for occult breast cancer. Ann Surg Oncol 2000;7(6):411–5.
51. Morris EA, Schwartz LH, Dershaw DD, et al. MR imaging of the breast in patients with occult primary breast carcinoma. Radiology 1997;205(2):437–40.
52. Orel SG, Weinstein SP, Schnall MD, et al. Breast MR imaging in patients with axillary node metastases and unknown primary malignancy. Radiology 1999;212(2):543–9.
53. Ko EY, Han BK, Shin JH, et al. Breast MRI for evaluating patients with metastatic axillary lymph node and initially negative mammography and sonography. Korean J Radiol 2007;8(5):382–9.
54. Varadarajan R, Edge SB, Yu J, et al. Prognosis of occult breast carcinoma presenting as isolated axillary nodal metastasis. Oncology 2006;71(5–6):456–9.
55. Sardanelli F, Melani E, Ottonello C, et al. Magnetic resonance imaging of the breast in characterizing positive or uncertain mammographic findings. Cancer Detect Prev 1998;22(1):39–42.
56. Lee CH, Smith RC, Levine JA, et al. Clinical usefulness of MR imaging of the breast in the evaluation of the problematic mammogram. AJR Am J Roentgenol 1999;173(5):1323–9.
57. Moy L, Elias K, Patel V, et al. Is breast MRI helpful in the evaluation of inconclusive mammographic findings? AJR Am J Roentgenol 2009;193(4):986–93.
58. Lehman CD, DeMartini W, Anderson BO, et al. Indications for breast MRI in the patient with newly diagnosed breast cancer. J Natl Compr Canc Netw 2009;7(2):193–201.

Comparison of Costs and Benefits of Breast Cancer Screening with Mammography, Ultrasonography, and MRI

Stephen Feig, MD

KEYWORDS

• Breast cancer • MRI • Mammography • Ultrasound

The cost-effectiveness of screening can be described using several different parameters: the *cost per breast cancer detected* is calculated by dividing the total cost of a screening program by the number of cancers detected. The program cost = (cost per mammogram + [cost × frequency of imaging workup for screen-detected abnormalities] + [cost × frequency of image-guided biopsy]) × number of women screened.

The *cost per breast cancer death averted* is calculated by (1) dividing screening program costs by the difference in breast cancer mortality between study and control groups found in randomized screening trials (RCTs), such as the Swedish Two-County Trial, or in service screening studies, such as the Swedish Seven-County Study[1,2] or (2) the expected differences in breast cancer deaths based on size and stage of detected tumors versus those in a comparable nonscreened population.

The *cost per year of life expectancy gained* is calculated by dividing the screening program costs by the expected number of years of life gained among screened women. The years of life gained through screening can be calculated by (1) subtracting the lifespan of patients with breast cancer in the control group from the lifespan of patients with breast cancer in the study group observed in RCT's or service screening studies or (2) expected gain in lifespan based on the size and stage of detected tumors versus those in comparable nonscreened population.

A version of this article was previously published as "Cost Effectiveness of Mammography, MRI, and Ultrasonography for Breast Cancer Screening," in *Radiologic Clinics* 48:5.
Department of Radiological Sciences, UC Irvine Medical Center, 101 The City Drive South, Orange, CA 92868, USA
E-mail address: sfeig@uci.edu

Obstet Gynecol Clin N Am 38 (2011) 179–196
doi:10.1016/j.ogc.2011.02.009
0889-8545/11/$ – see front matter © 2011 Elsevier Inc. All rights reserved.

obgyn.theclinics.com

A cost analysis of the US National Breast and Cervical Cancer Early Detection Program found that in 2003 and 2004, the median cost of screening mammography was $94 and the cost per cancer detected was $10,566. For cervical cancer, these costs were $56 and $13,340, respectively. This program provides screening for medically underserved low-income women aged 40 to 64 years for breast cancer and aged 18 to 64 years for cervical cancer.[3]

Screening program costs depend on screening protocols. Annual screening finds most cancers earlier than biennial screening but doubles the cost.[4] Screening with craniocaudal and mediolateral oblique (MLO) mammographic views detects 3% to 11% (mean 7%) more cancers but is costlier than screening using bilateral MLO views alone.[5]

Digital mammography detects more cancers in women younger than 50 years with dense breasts but is more expensive than conventional mammography.[6,7] Tosteson and colleagues[7] estimated that substitution of digital mammography for film mammography is not cost-effective, because Medicare reimbursement for screening with digital mammography is 60% more than film mammography ($135.29 vs $85.65), and overall detection rates are not increased except in women with dense breasts. However, restricting digital screening mammography to women with dense breasts is neither practical for a breast imaging facility nor acceptable to most patients.

SCREENING MAMMOGRAPHY

The cost per cancer detected is always lower in older populations, because screening detection rates parallel the natural cancer incidence, thus increasing with age. The cost per life saved and cost per year of life expectancy gained progressively decreases from age 40 years until age 70 years but then increases as a result of the lower normal life expectancy among older women. Assuming a 30% reduction in breast cancer mortality through annual screening mammography, Rosenquist and Lindfors[8] estimated that the cost per year of life expectancy saved was $26,000, $16,000, $15,000, $20,000, and $35,000 for women aged 40 to 49, 50 to 59, 60 to 69, 70 to 79, and 80 to 85 years at detection, respectively. Although population costs per year of life expectancy gained are higher for screening women in their 40s, the average woman with breast cancer detected by screening during that decade stands to gain more years of life expectancy than her older counterpart with breast cancer detected by screening during a later decade of life.

Many investigators have calculated the cost-effectiveness of screening women in their 40s. Their estimates have varied because of the different assumptions for benefits and costs and the different methods of calculation. Using data from the Breast Cancer Detection Demonstration Projects conducted in the United States in the 1970s, Moskowitz and Fox,[9,10] Eddy,[11] and Feig[12] independently derived estimates for the cost-effectiveness of screening women aged 40 to 49 years that were similar to or lower than those of Rosenquist and Lindfors. A study published by Salzmann and colleagues[13] in 1997 claiming that screening women aged 40 to 49 years is not cost-effective is no longer valid, because they used a 16% mortality reduction for screening women aged 40 to 49 years, which is too low.

Calculations by Rosenquist and Lindfors assumed a cost of $84 for a conventional mammogram in 1994 dollars. Current 2010 Medicare reimbursement is approximately $82 for conventional screening mammography and $130 for digital screening mammography. Recent service screening studies performed with conventional mammography have found a 40% to 45% mortality reduction for screened women aged 40 to 74 years.[2,14] However, even if the current costs per year of life expectancy saved are higher than those used by Rosenquist and Lindfors, they are still lower than the $100,000 per year of life threshold deemed to be acceptably cost-effective for other preventive medical procedures and tests.[15]

A subsequent study by Rosenquist and Lindfors estimated that annual screening mammography beginning at age 40 years and continuing until age 79 years would cost $18,800 per year of life expectancy saved.[16] The assumption for screening benefit in that study was that annual screening would reduce breast cancer deaths by 36% for cancers detected in women aged 40 to 49 years and by 45%, in women aged 50 to 79 years. Their estimate for the cost-effectiveness of screening mammography is in the same general range as that for other commonly accepted interventions, such as screening for cervical cancer and osteoporosis (**Table 1**). The cost per year of life gained from annual screening mammography is higher than that for screening for colorectal cancer but is much lower than that for the use of seat belts and airbags in automobiles.[17] Several other investigations found that annual and biennial screenings are cost-effective for all ages studied.[9,10,18,19] Annual screening is more effective but less cost-effective. Addition of computed-aided detection to the screening protocol increases the mean cost per year of life saved by 19% but is still within the accepted range for cost-effectiveness.[20]

COSTS OF SCREENING RECALL AND BIOPSY

In a low-cost screening project in Southern California in 1986 reported by Cyrlak,[21] the costs of screening mammograms accounted for less than one-third of total screening program costs, with diagnostic imaging workups, surgical consultations, and biopsies for benign disease representing the major induced costs of screening. In this study, 18% of women were recalled from screening for additional imaging workup or clinical evaluation. Among 72 biopsied patients, only 12 were found to have malignancy, that is, a biopsy positive predictive value (PPV) of 17% (12 of 72).

Table 1
Median cost per life-year saved for annual mammographic screening of women aged 40 to 79 years and other selected types of lifesaving interventions

Intervention	Median Cost per Year of Life Saved ($)
Colorectal screening	3000
Cholesterol screening	6000
Cervical cancer screening	12,000
Antihypertensive drugs	15,000
Osteoporosis screening	18,000
Mammography screening	18,800
Coronary artery bypass surgery	26,000
Automobile seat belts and air bags	32,000
Hormone replacement therapy	42,000
Renal dialysis	46,000
Heart transplant	54,000
Cholesterol treatment	154,000

Data on non-mammographic interventions *from* Tengs TO, Adams M, Pliskin J, et al. Five hundred life-saving interventions and their cost-effectiveness. Risk Anal 1995;15:369–90.

Cost-effectiveness estimate for screening mammography *from* Rosenquist CJ, Lindfors KK. Screening mammography beginning at age 40 years: a reappraisal of cost-effectiveness. Cancer 1998;82:2235–40.

Screening costs can be reduced without sacrificing early detection if radiologists achieve the clinical outcome values recommended by the US Agency for Health Care Policy and Research (now renamed the Agency for Health Care Research and Quality).[22] These desirable values include a screening recall rate of 10% or less and a PPV when biopsy is recommended (PPV$_2$) of 25% to 40%. These values are further described in the American College of Radiology (ACR) Breast Imaging Reporting and Database (BI-RADS) Atlas.[23] A recent survey of screening results at Breast Cancer Surveillance Consortium (BCSC) sites throughout the United States found a mean recall rate of 9.7% (12.3% on initial screen and 8.8% in subsequent screens). This means that nearly half of all sites had recall rates higher than the recommended upper limit of 10%. Results from BCSC sites are believed to represent practice throughout the country. BCSC sites also reported that their PPV$_2$ at screening was 25.0%, just at the lower limit of the recommended range.[24] Radiologists having clinical outcome values that differ substantially from the recommended values should consider additional training to modify their interpretive thresholds.[25]

Screen-detected lesions appropriately categorized as probably benign (BI-RADS 3) should have a less than 2% likelihood of malignancy. These lesions may be safely followed up at 6 months, 12 months, and annually thereafter, rather than biopsied. Adoption of this concept over the past 20 years has reduced the number of false-positive biopsy results, a potentially large component of screening costs.[26] False-positive callbacks for additional mammographic views and/or ultrasonography are another potentially large component of screening costs.

Widespread implementation in the United States of image-guided core biopsy instead of open surgical biopsy has occurred since 1990. At most facilities, these biopsies now represent of the majority for screen-detected lesions.[27–29] Costs of image-guided core biopsy are 16% to 33% of those for an open excisional biopsy.[30–37] Use of needle core biopsy instead of surgical biopsy can reduce the cost per year of life saved by screening by 23% ($20,770 to $15,934).[38]

In contrast with the screening program conducted in Southern California in 1986,[21] the one conducted in New Hampshire a decade later showed that 68% of its costs were from screening and only 32% of the costs were from consequent diagnostic imaging, biopsy, and surgical consultation.[39] This probably reflects a lower screening callback rate, substitution of short-term follow-up of probably benign lesions for biopsy, image-guided core biopsy instead of surgical biopsy for initial histologic diagnosis, and fewer surgical consults. Results from the 1996 to 2000 study of Poplack and colleagues[39] are similar to contemporary studies by Lidbrink and colleagues[40] and Elmore and colleagues[41] in which additional costs of evaluating false-positive results can add up to one-third of the total cost of screening all women.

Yet, even during the years 1996 to 2000, excisional biopsies represented 65% of all diagnostic costs versus 31% for stereotactic and ultrasound-guided biopsies.[29] It has been estimated that more than one million breast biopsies are performed in the United States yearly, but fewer than 25% prove to be malignant. Use of image-guided core biopsies instead of open surgical biopsies for all lesions would be equivalent to a cost reduction of about $1.5 billion.[42]

SCREENING MAMMOGRAPHY RESULTS, GUIDELINES, AND CONTROVERSIES: ROLE OF COST-EFFECTIVENESS

Screening controversies have been recurrent since 1975, when screening began to be widely used in the United States. With long-term follow-up, screening trials have demonstrated convincingly greater proof of benefit. Since 1997, annual screening for all women aged 40 years and older has been recommended by the American Cancer Society (ACS) and the ACR.[43,44] Currently, about 51% of all women in this age group report that they have had a mammogram in the past year and 67%, in the past 2 years.[45] The most recent screening controversy erupted in November 2009 with the publication of a series of papers in the Annals of Internal Medicine accompanied by issuance of new screening guidelines from the United States Preventive Services Task Force (USPSTF).[46–48]

The new USPSTF guidelines advise against any screening for women in their 40s except for those at very high risk.[46] Gross underestimation of the benefits for screening women in their 40s and unwarranted concern regarding callbacks and false-positive biopsy results in that age group were used as justification.[48] The USPSTF underestimated the mortality reduction for women offered screening in their 40s as 15%, rather than the 30% shown in the Swedish randomized trials.[49] More correctly, the benefit from service screening of women aged 40 to 49 years should be 48%, as found in the Swedish Two-County Study, 40%, in the British Columbia study, and/or 30%, in the study in 2 Northern Swedish counties.[2,14,50] The USPSTF then arbitrarily determined that the number needed to invite (NNI) to screening in their 40s to prevent one death from breast cancer was too small to justify screening average-risk women in that age group. Although monetary cost of screening was not mentioned per se in their report, it is clear that NNI is a code word for financial cost-effectiveness.

The USPSTF should not have included results from the National Breast Screening Study of Canada (NBSS) in the 40- to 49-year and 50- to 59-year age group estimates because of major problems in design and execution of the NBSS.[50] Because of a fatal flaw in the NBSS protocol, women presenting with late-stage breast cancer to screening centers were preferentially enrolled in the NBSS study group rather than being equally enrolled in study and control groups. This resulted in an excess of late-stage breast cancers and breast cancer deaths in the study group. Additionally, NBSS mammograms were often technically deficient, even by the standards of the 1980s, when the trial was conducted, a conclusion confirmed by numerous outside consultants invited by NBSS to evaluate mammographic image quality.[51] If the USPSTF had not included NBSS results in their meta-analysis, their calculated mortality reduction among 39- to 59-year-old women would have been 26% to 30% instead of 15%.

A second major change in screening recommendations was directed at women aged 50 to 75 years,[47] where the USPSTF recommended biennial instead of annual screening. Their rationale for less frequent screening of older women was their estimate that biennial screening could achieve 81% (range 67%–99%) of the benefit of annual screening while halving the number of mammograms and biopsies.[48] The USPSTF ignored other mathematical models, such as the one by Michaelson and colleagues,[52] which estimate that annual screening will double the benefit of biennial screening. Again, cost seems to be the unspoken rationale for their recommendations.

Reduced Treatment Costs Through Detection of Earlier Disease

It is well established that the costs of initial care, continuing care, and terminal care for patients with breast cancer increase according to the stage at diagnosis. Treatment and management costs become progressively greater for in situ, local, regional, and distant metastatic breast cancer.[53] A 4-year follow-up study by Legoretta and colleagues[54] of 200 women with newly diagnosed breast cancer in 1989 among 180,000 women enrolled in a health maintenance organization in Southeastern Pennsylvania found that the mean cumulative costs for stage 0, I, II, and stages III and IV were $18,900, $23,200, $28,800, and $55,000, respectively.[54] Of the total cohort of 200 patients, 116 (58%) were initially detected through mammographic screening. Among these screening-detected cancers, 74% (n = 86) were stage 0 or I; 24% (n = 28), stage II; and 2% (n = 2), stage III or IV. Among the 84 nonscreened patients with breast cancer, 31% (n = 26) were stage 0 or I; 52% (n = 44), stage II; and 17% (n = 14), stage III or IV. The mean cumulative treatment costs over 4 years were $31,000 for patients with breast cancer who had not undergone screening and $23,000 for those who had.

Several studies have compared the cost of screening with the savings from decreased treatment costs. In a Norwegian service screening program, breast cancer mortality was reduced by 30% among women offered screening biennially between ages 50 and 69 years. Norum[55] estimated that 33% of the screening costs were offset by the consequent lower treatment costs. Another screening program in Nijmegan and Utrecht in the Netherlands also offered biennial screening to women aged 50 to 70 years beginning in the late 1980s.[56] Breast cancer deaths were initially reduced by 12% at an attendance rate of 70%. Van der Maas and colleagues[19] also found that 33% of the cost of screening was offset by the decreased need for advanced care. In a longer-term follow-up analysis, de Koning and colleagues[57] found that breast cancer mortality reduction was 23%. After program start-up costs had ended, as much as 47% of the remaining annual program cost was offset by the lower cost of treatment.[57–59]

A study at the Jackson Memorial Hospital/University of Miami by Zavertnik and colleagues[60] compared stage of disease, 5-year survival rates, and treatment costs before and after implementation of a screening mammography program in Dade County Florida in 1987. Comparing 1990 with 1983 to 1988, the frequency of in situ disease increased from 2.7% to 33.3% and local disease, from 30.4% to 38.1%; whereas regional disease decreased from 46.2% to 28.6% and distant metastatic disease, from 20.7% to 0%. The 5-year survival rate increased from 50% to 74%. Treatment costs were $5000 per case for in situ, local, and regional disease and $80,000 per case for distant and recurrent disease. The total cost for screening and treatment in the early detection program was $2,424,532. The estimated cost of treatment without the screening program was $2,594,029. Thus, the investigators calculated that the screening program saved $169,497 ($2,594,029 − $2,424,532), a savings of $14.28 per mammogram performed or $2872.83 per patient whose breast cancer was diagnosed and treated. Even greater improvement in stage at diagnosis was reported after 1990, equivalent to savings of $46.89 per mammogram performed or $9745.83 per patient whose cancer was diagnosed and treated.

In a similar type study, Glenn[61] used Brooke Army Medical Center (BAMC) patient data and Department of Defense Tumor Registry data to compare breast cancer staging distribution at BAMC during the period before 1980 when there was no screening and 1994 to 1995 when there was increased screening. Costs of treatment for each stage were calculated using 1994 current procedural terminology and diagnosis-related group codes in the BAMC Medical Expense Reporting System (MEPRS). A theoretical population of 100,000 women with 500 breast cancers per year was assumed. The total cost of breast care, including screening, workup, diagnosis, and treatment, was $16.6 million for no screening (pre-1980) versus $10.5 million for the 1994 to 1995 screening years. The total cost per patient was $166 for no screening (pre-1980) versus $105 for the 1994 to 1995 screening years. The investigator concluded that cost-efficient screening involves high front-end costs, but these are more than offset in the long run by dollars saved through lower treatment costs.

Using breast cancer detection rates and mortality reduction results from the Health Insurance Plan of New York (HIP) randomized trial, which screened women aged 40 to 64 years with annual mammography and clinical examination in the 1960s, Moskowitz[62] applied 1987 screening and treatment costs to compare the total costs for 65,000 screens performed at HIP versus no screening.[11] Screening costs included mammography, time off from work to attend screening, and induced costs, such as ultrasonography, additional mammography, aspiration, and false-positive biopsy results. When the costs avoided were limited to those for treatment of more advanced disease for the 37 women whose lives were saved through screening, these costs were $2,220,000 compared with screening costs of $4,072,200. However, when the avoided costs also included costs for short-term disability, long-term disability, and employee replacement, the total cost of not screening was $5,570,160, thus, far exceeding the costs of screening. Therefore, the net effect on a health-care system engendered by the HIP screening program using 1987 costs would be a gain of about $1,497,960 ($5,570,160 − $4,072,200). Strictly speaking, cost-effectiveness compares the costs for a given intervention with the costs of no intervention.[62] When the ratio of the cost of the intervention is less than one, it is clearly cost-effective. The cost-effectiveness ratio calculated by Moskowitz[62] for HIP screening was 0.73. Strictly speaking, the cost per death averted and the cost per year of life gained are measures of cost-benefit rather than cost-effectiveness. Using 1987 costs, Moskowitz found that the cost per year of life saved in HIP was $3770.[11]

MAGNETIC RESONANCE IMAGING SCREENING OF VERY HIGH-RISK WOMEN: RESULTS AND GUIDELINES

Unlike mammography, no randomized trial has ever been conducted to evaluate whether magnetic resonance imaging (MRI) screening can reduce breast cancer mortality. However, since 2004, 9 nonoverlapping series with a total of 4485 very high-risk women screened with mammography and MRI found that 36% (70 of 192) of cancers were detected by mammography and an additional 56% (108 of 192) were identified only by MRI for a combined screening sensitivity of 92.7% (4157 of 4485).[63–71] Eligibility criteria for these trials were largely a projected lifetime risk of 20% to 25% or the presence of BRCA1 or 2 mutation in the patient or a first-degree relative.[72]

On the basis of these trial results, in 2007, the ACS recommended annual screening MRI as a supplement to annual screening mammography for women at very high risk of breast cancer.[73]

These included women who:

- BRCA1 or 2 mutation or are untested first-degree relatives of a BRCA carrier
- lifetime risk of 20% to 25% or more using a breast cancer risk model, such as BRCAPRO(BRCA probability), Tyrer-Cuzick, BOADICEA(Breast and Ovarian Analysis of Disease Incidence and Carrier Estimation Algorithm), Gail, or Claus.

Based on expert consensus opinion, the ACS also recommended annual mammography and annual MRI screening for the following women:

- History of receiving radiation to the chest between age 10 and 30 years, usually for treatment of Hodgkin disease
- Those with Li-Fraumeni, Cowden, or Bannayen-Riley-Ruvalcaba syndromes or their first-degree relatives.

The ACS found insufficient evidence to recommend or not recommend annual MRI for women having a lifetime risk of 15% to 20% or those at increased risk because of biopsy-proven lobular carcinoma in situ (LCIS); atypical lobular hyperplasia (ALH); atypical ductal hyperplasia (ADH); heterogeneously or extremely dense breasts on mammography; or their personal history of invasive carcinoma or in situ ductal carcinoma (DCIS). The ACS recommended against screening MRI for women at less than 15% lifetime risk.

In 2008, the National Comprehensive Cancer Network recommended that women with BRCA1 or 2 mutation begin screening MRI at age 25 years.[74]

In 2010, the Society of Breast Imaging and the American College of Radiology made the following recommendations for screening high-risk women[75]:

- BRCA1 or 2 carriers or their first-degree relatives should begin annual mammography and annual MRI by age 30 years but not before 25 years
- Women with a 20% or higher lifetime risk of breast cancer should begin annual mammography and annual MRI by age 30 years (but not before 20 years) or 10 years before the age that their youngest affected first-degree relative developed breast cancer, whichever is later.
- Women having a history of chest irradiation between ages 10 and 30 years should begin annual mammography and annual MRI eight years after treatment but not before age 25 years.
- For women with a history of breast cancer (invasive cancer or DCIS), ovarian cancer, biopsy-proven lobular neoplasia (ALH or LCIS), or ADH, annual mammography and annual MRI should also be considered from the time of diagnosis.

MRI SCREENING OF VERY HIGH-RISK WOMEN: COST-EFFECTIVENESS

Several studies have evaluated the cost-effectiveness of screening MRI. Plevritis and colleagues[76] estimated that the cost per quality-adjusted life year (QALY) for annual screening with mammography and MRI relative to screening with mammography alone between ages 35 and 54 years was $55,420 for women with a BRCA1 mutation and $130,695, for BRCA2. For women with dense breasts, estimated cost per QALY was $41,183 for BRCA1 carriers and $98,454 for BRCA2. Higher cancer rates and more aggressive cancers in BRCA1 compared with BRCA2 carriers and lower sensitivity of mammography in women with dense breasts can explain these differences.

A recent study by Lee and colleagues[77] compared 3 different annual screening strategies starting at age 25 years for a BRCA1 carrier: combined screening with mammography and MRI, MRI alone, and mammography alone. Compared with an estimated 533 breast cancer deaths among 1000 women having clinical surveillance alone, the estimated number of breast cancer deaths was 446 for mammography alone, 438 for MRI alone, and 415 for MRI and mammography combined. Although combined screening was the most effective in reducing deaths, it had the slightly higher cost at $110,973 per QALY compared with $108,641 and $100,336 per QALY for screening with MRI alone and mammography alone, respectively.

MRI SCREENING OF MODERATELY HIGH-RISK WOMEN: COST-EFFECTIVENESS

Using results from the Magnetic Resonance Imaging Breast Screening Study (MARIBS) conducted in the UK, Griebsch and colleagues[78] found that the incremental cost of adding MRI screening to mammographic screening for women having a 50% likelihood of BRCA1 or 2 was $50,911 per cancer detected. For known mutation carriers, the cost was $27,544 per cancer detected. A further analysis of the UK MRI screening data found that the incremental cost of screening 40- to 49-year-old women with mammography and MRI versus mammography alone was $14,005 per QALY for a BRCA carrier having a 31% ten-year breast cancer risk. For 40- to 49-year-old non-BRCA carriers, the cost per QALY was $53,320 and $96,379 for those with a 12% and 6% ten-year risk, respectively. For 30- to 39-year-old women, the incremental cost was $24,275 for BRCA1 carriers (10-year risk of 11%) and $70,054 for high-risk non-BRCA carriers (10-year risk of 5%).[78] These estimates were based on costs within the UK National Health Service. Current UK policy is to offer screening MRI to women aged 30 to 39 years at familial risk, having a 10-year risk of more than 8%. For women aged 40 to 49 years, screening MRI is offered to those at a 10-year risk of 20% or more. For women aged 40 to 49 years with dense breasts having lower mammographic sensitivity, screening MRI is offered to those with a 10-year risk of 12% or more.[79]

A model to evaluate the cost-effectiveness of screening high-risk women with MRI and mammography versus mammography alone was developed by Taneja and colleagues.[80] These investigators estimated that among 10,000 women age 40 years with BRCA1 or 2 mutations, 400 (4% prevalence) would have clinically undiagnosed breast cancer. Among these, 361 would be detected by MRI and mammography combined, 290 by MRI alone, and 160 by mammography alone. For these women, the incremental cost per QALY gained through screening with MRI and mammography versus mammography alone was estimated at $25,270. For non-BRCA women with an annual breast cancer prevalence of 3%, 2%, or 1%, the incremental cost per QALY gained was calculated as $73,813, $154,045, and $315,210, respectively. The authors concluded that MRI is cost-effective for BRCA carriers and also for other very high-risk women, albeit at the higher end ($100,000) of the generally accepted range for those with a prevalence of 2.5% to 3.0%.

IMPACT OF RISK ASSESSMENT MODELS AND FUTURE TECHNICAL ADVANCES ON COST-EFFECTIVENESS OF MRI SCREENING

Because the cost of MRI is more than $1000 compared with about $100 for mammography, accurate determination of individual breast cancer risk is essential for a cost-effective MRI screening program. By age 70 years, the lifetime risk of breast cancer is 65% for BRCA1 carriers and 45% for BRCA2 carriers[81] compared with a cumulative lifetime risk of 12% by age 80 years for a woman with no known risk factors.[82] All current risk models are inaccurate for predicting breast cancer risk for the vast majority of women, who are non-BRCA carriers. The prevalence of BRCA1 mutations is estimated to be between 1:500 and 1:1000 in the general population.[83] The ACS estimated the lifetime risk for 5 hypothetical women using 3 risk models: BRCAPRO, Claus, and Tyrer-Cuzick to determine whether they met the 20% or greater lifetime risk level set by ACS MRI screening guidelines.[73] Among them, 2 women qualified according to only one of the 3 models; 2, according to two of the 3 models; and only one, according to all 3 models.[73] According to Amir and colleagues,[84] risk models may underestimate risk by as much as 50% in observed populations. Using women from their own practice, these investigators found that the ratios of expected to observed breast cancers were 0.48 for the Gail model, 0.56 for the Claus model, 0.49 for the Ford model, and 0.81 for the Tyrer-Cuzick model. Although the Tyrer-Cuzick model was more accurate than the other 3 models, it underestimated risk by 19%.[84]

Compared with a woman with no known risk factor, the relative risk of developing breast cancer is increased in women with: a personal history of breast cancer

(8–10x overall; 3–4x for a second primary)[85,86]; two or more family members with breast cancer (2.9x)[82]; a mother diagnosed before age 50 years (2.4x)[87]; a sister diagnosed before age 50 years (3.2x)[87]; a personal history of biopsy-proven LCIS (8–12x),[88] ADH (4–5x),[89] or ALH (3x)[90]; and dense breasts on mammography (4–6x).[91] Development of a single model to more accurately predict breast cancer risk through incorporation of all of these family and personal risk factors is much needed. Conducting clinical studies to determine MRI-only detection rates for women in the 15% to 20% lifetime risk group is also needed. Such data could be used to better determine the cost-effectiveness of MRI for each projected risk level. It has also been suggested by Berg[92] that 10-year risk may be more accurate than lifetime risk.

In the future, evolving MRI techniques, such as diffusion-weighted imaging, spectroscopy, and noncontrast perfusion imaging might reduce examination time and eliminate the need for intravenous contrast injection, so that breast MRI could be performed faster and at lower cost.[93] If successful, these techniques would improve the cost-effectiveness of MRI and allow cost-effective screening of greater numbers of women.

SCREENING ULTRASONOGRAPHY: TARGET POPULATIONS

Among the 9 series of very high-risk women screened with MRI and mammography, 4 also included ultrasonography. These 4 series found that the sensitivity of mammography and ultrasonography combined was only 52%, compared with a 92.7% sensitivity for mammography and MRI combined.[64,67–69] This observation that the sensitivity of MRI is much higher than that of ultrasonography is substantiated by the clinical experience that most MRI-detected cancers cannot be localized for ultrasound-guided biopsy but require MRI-guided biopsy instead.[94]

The main indication for screening ultrasonography is women with dense fibroglandular breast tissue in whom mammographic detection rates are lower.

Although ultrasonography is a less sensitive screening examination than MRI, combined screening with mammography and ultrasonography has been found to substantially increase detection rates beyond those from mammography alone. The lower sensitivity of mammography for cancer detection in dense breasts first noted in the 1970s[95] persists to a lesser degree in more recent studies.[96–101] Dense breasts, usually defined as breasts having 50% or greater dense tissue, are more common among younger women. The prevalence of dense breasts among women age 30 to 39, 40 to 49, 50 to 59, and 60 to 69 was found to be 62%, 56%, 38%, and 27%, respectively by Stomper and colleagues.[102] Thus, the number of women with dense breasts who might benefit from supplementary screening with breast ultrasonography far exceeds the estimated 1.4 million American women who would qualify for supplementary screening with breast MRI according to ACS MRI screening guidelines.[73]

NONBLINDED ULTRASONOGRAPHIC SCREENING TRIALS

Between 1995 and 2003, 42,836 women with generally dense breast tissue were screened with mammography and ultrasonography using hand-held high-resolution transducers (7.5–10.0 MHz) in 6 published series.[103–110] Interpretations were nonblinded to those of the other modality. A review of these studies by Feig[111] found that cancer detection rates with ultrasonography alone ranged from 2.7 to 9.0 per 1000 (mean = 3.5 per 1000). Mean tumor size was 1.0 cm for ultrasonography-only lesions. PPVs for biopsies and aspirations performed by ultrasonography alone ranged from 6.6% to 18.0% (mean = 11.4%). For 4 series that separately analyzed results for core biopsies of solid lesions, PPV for ultrasonography alone ranged from 11.8% to 20.5%. The detection rate of 3.5 per 1000 for ultrasonography alone is extremely encouraging because at BCSC Centers considered generally representative of clinical practice in the United States, the detection rate at mammographic screening is 4.4 per 1000 examinations.[24] The mean tumor size of 1.0 cm for ultrasonography-only cancers is also encouraging because it more than fulfills the US Agency for Health Care Policy and Research (AHCPR) recommendation that 30% or more of mammographic screening-detected cancers be minimal (<1 cm invasive or DCIS) and that 50% or more be Stage 0 or I.[112] However, because AHCPR recommends a PPV_2 of 25% to 40% for screening mammography, the frequency of false-positive biopsies for ultrasonography-only lesions is greater than that expected for screening mammography.[112,113]

BLINDED ULTRASONOGRAPHIC SCREENING TRIALS

Because nonblinded studies may be subject to reader bias, the ACR Imaging Network (ACRIN) initiated ACRIN Trial 6666 to determine if results from the prior 6 nonblinded ultrasonographic screening studies could be duplicated under a more scientifically rigorous protocol. Radiologist readers of mammography and ultrasonography were each masked to results from the other modality. Following initial screening of 2809 very high-risk women having dense breasts, Berg and colleagues[114] diagnosed 41 cancers: 12 on mammography alone, 12 on ultrasonography alone, 8 on mammography and ultrasonography, and 9 on neither modality. The diagnostic yield was 7.6 cancers per 1000 women on mammography versus 11.8 cancers per 1000 women for combined screening with mammography and ultrasonography, for a supplementary yield of 4.2 cancers per 1000 women. Although the 95% confidence interval was wide, 1.1 to 7.2 per 1000, the results of this study suggest that among women with dense breasts, supplementary ultrasonographic screening is associated with a 50% increase in cancer detection. Median size of ultrasonography-detected cancers was 1 cm. The study also confirms findings from prior studies that false-positive biopsy rates are higher on ultrasonography than on mammography. At ACRIN 6666, the PPV_2 was 8.9% for ultrasonography versus 22.6% for mammography and 11.2% for combined ultrasonographic and mammographic screening.

The value of screening ultrasonography was further corroborated in another blinded study of hand-held ultrasonography by Corsetti and colleagues[115] in Italy. An initial negative mammographic assessment was confirmed at subsequent review by 4 internal radiologists and an external expert radiologist. Among 9157 women with negative mammographic assessments and dense breasts, ultrasonography alone found 4.0 cancers per 1000 women. The overall incremental cancer detection rate for ultrasonography was 20.6% for all women, 41.3% for those younger than 50 years, and 13.5% for those older than 50 years. This study suggests that the most cost-effective strategy would result from using ultrasonography as a supplementary screening modality in younger women with dense breasts. Among cancers detected by ultrasonography alone by Corsetti and colleagues, 65% were less than 1 cm and 27% were 1 to 2 cm. The proportion of minimal cancers (invasive <1 cm or DCIS) was higher for detection by ultrasonography alone than for mammographic detection: 65% versus 36%. PPV for ultrasonography-only biopsies was 37.5%, much higher than in the other ultrasonography screening studies. Corsetti and colleagues estimated that the cost per cancer detected by ultrasonography alone was $18,900 to $19,760, higher than the cost of $6350 per mammography-detected cancer. This higher cost of ultrasonography is because it increased the detection rate by 20.6% while approximately doubling the overall cost of screening.

AUTOMATED ULTRASONOGRAPHIC SCREENING

The length of time for the US screening examination is another limitation and was clocked at 19 minutes in the ACRIN trial, moderately higher than the estimated examination times in other studies of ultrasonographic screening performed using hand-held transducers. Thus, total radiologist time for performance, interpretation, and report dictation for ultrasonographic screening could be 25 to 30 minutes. By comparison, the time for interpretation of screening mammography was measured as 5 minutes by Enzmann and colleagues.[116] Screening with hand-held ultrasonography performed by a radiologist may be a time-consuming and expensive endeavor and would lose money for a facility at the current Medicare reimbursement rate of $80 for diagnostic ultrasonography. More importantly, neither Medicare nor most other insurers currently pay for screening ultrasonography. Radiologist staff shortages are another consideration, because a radiologist may be able to complete only 2 to 3 hand-held ultrasonographic screening examinations per hour versus interpretation of 20 to 50 screening mammograms per hour depending on whether automatic reporting systems are used.

One way to decrease the cost of breast ultrasonographic screening would be through the use of an automated whole-breast ultrasound scanner (ABUS). Potential advantages would be elimination of a radiologist or even an ultrasonography technologist to perform the study, standardization of an examination that is notoriously operator-dependant, and reduction in examination time. Several automated ultrasound scanners have been developed and are under clinical investigation.[117] In one study of automated breast ultrasonography, Kelly and colleagues[118] screened 6425 women with dense breasts and/or elevated risk of breast cancer. In this nonblinded study, ultrasonography alone found a prevalence of 3.6 cancers per 1000 women, similar to that in studies performed with hand-held units. Among cancers detected by ultrasonography alone, 64% were 1 cm or less and 91% were 2 cm or less, generally smaller sizes than found with mammographic screening at the BCSC.[24] Biopsy PPV for ABUS was 38.4%, higher than that for the ACRIN trial and similar to the 39.0% PPV for mammography in the ABUS population. The use of ABUS as a supplementary screening modality doubled the cancer detection rate from 3.6 per 1000 for mammography alone to 7.2 per 1000 for combined screening. At these incremental detection rates and at a cost of $300 per screening with ultrasonographic examination used by the investigators, ABUS would be only one-third as cost-effective as mammography but still within the generally acceptable range for cost-effectiveness and currently more cost-effective than MRI for most populations.

SUMMARY

Screening mammography performed annually on all women beginning at age 40 years has reduced breast cancer deaths by 30% to 50%. The cost per year of life saved is well within the range for other commonly accepted medical interventions. Various studies have estimated that reduction in treatment costs through early screening detection may be 30% to 100% or more of the cost of screening. MRI screening is also cost-effective for very high-risk women, such as BRCA carriers, and others at 20% or greater lifetime risk. Further studies are needed to determine whether MRI is cost-effective for those at moderately high (15%–20%) lifetime risk. Future technical advances could make MRI more cost-effective than it is today. Automated whole breast ultrasonography will probably prove cost-effective as a supplement to mammography for women with dense breasts.

REFERENCES

1. Tabar L, Vitak B, Chen H-H, et al. The Swedish Two County Trial twenty years later. Radiol Clin North Am 2000;38:625–52.
2. Tabar L, Yen M-F, Vitak B, et al. Mammography service screening and mortality in breast cancer patients: 20-year follow-up before and after introduction of screening. Lancet 2003;361:1405–10.
3. Ekwueme DU, Gardner JG, Subramanian S, et al. Cost analysis of the National Breast and Cervical Cancer Early Detection Program, selected states, 2003–2004. Cancer 2008;112:626–35.
4. Feig SA. Increased benefit from shorter screening mammography intervals for women ages 40–49 years. Cancer 1997;80:2035–9.
5. Feig SA. Estimation of currently attainable benefit from mammographic screening of women aged 40–49 years. Cancer 1995;75:2412–9.
6. Pisano ED, Gatsonis C, Hendrick E, et al. Diagnostic performance of digital versus film mammography for breast-cancer screening. N Engl J Med 2005; 353:1773–83.
7. Tosteson AN, Stout NK, Fryback DG, et al. Cost-effectiveness of digital mammography in breast cancer screening. Ann Intern Med 2008;148:1–10.
8. Rosenquist CJ, Lindfors KK. Screening mammography in women aged 40–49 years: analysis of cost-effectiveness. Radiology 1994;191:647–50.
9. Moskowitz M, Fox SH. Cost analysis of aggressive breast cancer screening. Radiology 1979;130:253–6.
10. Moskowitz M. Costs of screening for breast cancer. Radiol Clin North Am 1987; 25:1031–7.
11. Eddy DM. Screening for breast cancer. Ann Intern Med 1989;111:389–99.
12. Feig SA. Mammographic screening of women aged 40–49 years: benefit, risk, and cost considerations. Cancer 1995;76:2097–106.
13. Salzmann P, Kerlikowske K, Phillips K. Cost-effectiveness of screening mammography of women aged 40–49 years of age. Ann Intern Med 1997; 127:955–65.
14. Coldman A, Phillips N, Warren L, et al. Breast cancer mortality after screening mammography in British Columbia women. Int J Cancer 2006; 120:1076–80.
15. Gold M, Siegel J, Russell L, et al. Cost-effectiveness in health and medicine. New York: Oxford University Press; 1996.
16. Rosenquist CJ, Lindfors KK. Screening mammography beginning at age 40 years: a reappraisal of cost-effectiveness. Cancer 1998;82:2235–40.
17. Tengs TO, Adams M, Pliskin J, et al. Five hundred life-saving interventions and their cost-effectiveness. Risk Anal 1995;15:369–90.
18. Brown ML. Sensitivity analysis in the cost-effectiveness of breast cancer screening. Cancer 1992;69:1963–7.
19. Van der Maas PJ, de Koning HJ, Van Inveld M, et al. The cost-effectiveness of breast cancer screening. Int J Cancer 1989;43:1055–60.
20. Lindfors KK, McGahan MC, Rosenquist CJ, et al. Computer aided detection: a cost-effective study. Radiol 2006;238:710–7.
21. Cyrlak D. Induced costs of low-cost screening mammography. Radiology 1988; 168:661–3.
22. Bassett LW, Hendrick RG, Bassford TL, et al. Clinical practice guidelines number 13: quality determinants of mammography. Rockwell (MD): US Department of Health and Human Services; 1999. p. 83.

23. D'Orsi CJ, Bassett LW, Berg WA, et al. Breast imaging reporting and data system: ACR BI-RADS. 4th edition. Reston (VA): American College of Radiology; 2003. p. 229–51.
24. Rosenberg RD, Yankaskas BC, Abraham LA, et al. Performance benchmarks for screening mammography. Radiology 2006;241:55–66.
25. Carney PA, Sickles EA, Monsees B, et al. Identifying minimally acceptable interpretive performance criteria for screening mammography. Radiology 2010;255: 354–61.
26. Leung JWT, Sickles EA. The probably benign assessment. Radiol Clin North Am 2007;45:773–90.
27. March DE, Raslavicus A, Coughlin BF, et al. Use of core biopsy in the United States. Am J Roentgenol 1997;169:697–701.
28. Zannis VJ, Aliano KM. The evolving practice pattern of the breast surgeon with disappearance of open biopsy for nonpalpable lesions. Am J Surg 1998;176: 525–8.
29. Crowe JP, Rim A, Patrick R, et al. A prospective review of the decline of excisional breast biopsy. Am J Surg 2002;184:353–5.
30. Yim JH, Barton P, Weber B, et al. Mammographically detected breast cancer: benefits of stereotactic core versus wire localization biopsy. Ann Surg 1996; 223:688–700.
31. Pitre B, Baron PL, Baron LF, et al. Efficacy of stereotactic needle biopsy in the evaluation of mammographic abnormalities. Surg Forum 1995;46:625–7.
32. Schmidt RA. Stereotactic breast biopsy. CA Cancer J Clin 1994;44:172–91.
33. Howisey RL, Acheson MBG, Rowbotham RK, et al. A comparison of Medicare reimbursement and results for various imaging-guided breast biopsy techniques. Am J Surg 1997;173:395–8.
34. Lind DS, Minter R, Steinbach B, et al. Stereotactic core biopsy reduces the reexcision rate and the cost of mammographically detected cancer. J Surg Res 1998;78:23–6.
35. Rubin E, Mennemeyer ST, Desmond RA, et al. Reducing the cost of diagnosis of breast cancer. Cancer 2001;91:324–32.
36. Cross MJ, Evans WP, Peters GN, et al. Stereotactic breast biopsy as an alternative to open excisional biopsy. Ann Surg Oncol 1995;2:195–200.
37. Hillner BE, Bear HD, Fajardo LL. Estimating the cost-effectiveness of stereotactic biopsy for nonpalpable breast abnormalities: a decision analysis model. Acad Radiol 1996;3:351–60.
38. Lindfors KK, Rosenquist CJ. Needle core biopsy guided with mammography: a study of cost-effectiveness. Radiology 1994;190:217–22.
39. Poplack SP, Carney PA, Weiss JE, et al. Screening mammography: costs and use of screening-related services. Radiology 2005;234:79–85.
40. Lidbrink E, Elfving J, Frisell J, et al. Neglected aspects of false positive findings of mammography in breast cancer screening: analysis of false positive cases from the Stockholm trial. BMJ 1996;312:273–6.
41. Elmore JG, Barton MB, Moceri VM, et al. Ten-year risk of false positive screening mammograms and clinical breast examinations. N Engl J Med 1998;338:1089–96.
42. Nields MW. Cost-effectiveness of image-guided core needle biopsy versus surgery in diagnosing breast cancer. Acad Radiol 1996;3(Suppl 1):S138–40.
43. Smith RA, Saslow D, Sawyer KA, et al. American Cancer Society guidelines for breast cancer screening: update 2003. CA Cancer J Clin 2003;53:141–69.
44. Feig SA, D'Orsi CJ, Hendrick RE, et al. American College of Radiology Guidelines for breast cancer screening. AJR Am J Roentgenol 1998;171:29–33.

45. American Cancer Society. Cancer prevention and early detection facts and figures 2009. Atlanta (GA): American Cancer Society; 2009.
46. US Preventive Services Task Force. Screening for breast cancer: US preventive services task force recommendation statement. Ann Intern Med 2009;151:716–26.
47. Nelson HD, Tyne K, Naik A, et al. Screening for breast cancer: an update for the US preventive services task force. Ann Intern Med 2009;151:727–37.
48. Mandelblatt JS, Cronin KA, Bailey S, et al. Effects of mammography screening under different screening schedules: model estimates of potential benefits and harms. Ann Intern Med 2009;151:738–47.
49. Hendrick RE, Smith RA, Rutledge JH, et al. Benefit of screening mammography in women ages 40–49:a new meta-analysis of randomized controlled trials. J Natl Cancer Inst Monogr 1997;22:87–92.
50. Jonsson H, Bordas P, Wallin H, et al. Service screening with mammography in Northern Sweden: effects on breast cancer mortality annual updates. J Med Screen 2007;1:87–93.
51. Kopans DB, Feig SA. The Canadian National Breast Screening Study: a critical review. AJR Am J Roentgenol 1993;161:755–60.
52. Michaelson JS, Halpern E, Kopans DB. Breast cancer: computer simulation method for estimating optimal intervals for screening. Radiology 1999;212:551–60.
53. Taplin SH, Barlow W, Urban N, et al. Stage, age, comorbidity, and direct costs of colon, prostate, and breast cancer care. J Natl Cancer Inst 1995;87:417–26.
54. Legorreta AP, Brooks RJ, Liebowitz AN, et al. Costs of breast cancer treatment: a 4-year longitudinal study. Arch Intern Med 1996;156:2197–201.
55. Norum J. Breast cancer screening by mammography in Norway. Is it cost effective? Ann Oncol 1999;10:197–203.
56. Otto SJ, Fracheboud J, Looman CW, et al. Initiation of population-based mammography screening in Dutch municipalities and effect on breast cancer mortality: a systematic review. Lancet 2003;361:1411–7.
57. de Koning HJ, van Ineveld BM, van Oortmarssen GJ, et al. Breast cancer screening and cost-effectiveness; policy alternatives, quality of life considerations and the possible impact of uncertain factors. Int J Cancer 1991;49:531–7.
58. de Koning HJ, van Ineveld BM, de Haes JC, et al. Advanced breast cancer and its prevention by screening. Br J Cancer 1992;65:950–5.
59. de Koning HJ, Coebergh JW, van Dongen JA. Is mass screening for breast cancer cost-effective? Eur J Cancer 1996;32A(11):1835–9.
60. Zavertnik JJ, McCoy CB, Robinson DS, et al. Cost-effective management of breast cancer. Cancer 1992;69:1979–84.
61. Glenn ME. Can treatment dollars saved through earlier breast cancer diagnosis offset increased costs of mammography screening? The BAMC experience. Radiology 1997;205(P):142–3.
62. Moskowitz M. Cost-benefit determinations in screening mammography. Cancer 1987;60:1680–3.
63. Kriege M, Brekelmans CT, Boetes C, et al. Efficacy of MRI and mammography for breast cancer screening in women with a familial or genetic predisposition. N Engl J Med 2004;351:427–37.
64. Kuhl CK, Schrading S, Leutner CC, et al. Mammography, breast ultrasound, and magnetic resonance imaging for surveillance of women at high familial risk for breast cancer. J Clin Oncol 2005;23:8469–76.
65. Leach MO, Boggis CR, Dixon AK, et al. Screening with magnetic resonance imaging and mammography of a UK population at high familial risk of breast

cancer: a prospective multicentre cohort study (MARIBS). Lancet 2005;365: 1769–78.

66. Lehman CD, Blume JD, Weatherall P, et al. Screening women at high risk for breast cancer with mammography and magnetic resonance imaging. Cancer 2005;103:1898–905.

67. Sardanelli F, Podo F, D'Agnollo G, et al. Multicenter comparative multimodality surveillance of women at genetic-familial high risk for breast cancer (HIBCRIT study); interim results. Radiology 2007;242:698–715.

68. Warner E, Plewes DB, Hill KA, et al. Surveillance of BRCA1 and BRCA2 mutation carriers with magnetic resonance imaging, ultrasound, mammography, and clinical breast examination. JAMA 2004;292:1317–25.

69. Lehman CD, Issacs C, Schnall MD, et al. Cancer yield of mammography, MRI and US in high-risk women: prospective multi-institution breast cancer screening study. Radiology 2007;244:381–8.

70. Hagen AI, Kvistad KA, Maehle L, et al. Sensitivity of MRI versus conventional screening in the diagnosis of BRCA-associated breast cancer in a national prospective series. Breast 2007;16:367–74.

71. Hartman AR, Daniel BL, Kurian AW, et al. Breast magnetic resonance image screening and ductal lavage in women at high genetic risk for breast carcinoma. Cancer 2004;100:479–89.

72. Warner E, Messersmith H, Causer P, et al. Systematic review: using magnetic resonance imaging to screen for breast cancer. Ann Intern Med 2008;148: 671–9.

73. Saslow D, Boetes C, Burke W, et al. American Cancer Society guidelines for breast screening with MRI as and adjunct to mammography. CA Cancer J Clin 2007;57:75–89.

74. Bevers TB, Anderson BO, Bonaccio E, et al. Breast cancer screening and diagnosis. J Natl Compr Canc Netw 2009;7:1060–96.

75. Lee CH, Dershaw DD, Kopans D, et al. Breast cancer screening with imaging: recommendations from the Society of Breast Imaging and the ACR on the use of mammography, breast MRI, breast ultrasound, and other technologies for the detection of clinically occult breast cancer. J Am Coll Radiol 2010;7:18–27.

76. Plevritis SK, Kurian AW, Sigal BM, et al. Cost-effectiveness of screening BRCA 1/2 mutation carriers with breast magnetic resonance imaging. JAMA 2006;295: 2374–84.

77. Lee JM, McMahon PM, Kong CY, et al. Cost-effectiveness of breast MRI imaging and screen-film mammography for screening BRCA 1 gene mutation carriers. Radiology 2010;254:793–800.

78. Griebsch I, Brown J, Boggis C, et al. Cost-effectiveness of screening with contrast enhanced magnetic resonance imaging versus x-ray mammography of women at high familial risk of breast cancer. Br J Cancer 2006;95:801–10.

79. National Institute for Clinical Excellence (NICE), National Collaborating Centre for Primary Care. Familial breast cancer – the classification and care of women at risk of familial breast cancer in primary, secondary, and tertiary care. Available at: http://www.nice.org.uk. Accessed January 5, 2010.

80. Taneja C, Edelsberg J, Weycker D, et al. Cost effectiveness of breast cancer screening with contrast- enhanced MRI in high-risk women. J Am Coll Radiol 2009;6:171–9.

81. Easton DF, Ford D, Bishop DT. Breast and ovarian cancer incidence in BRCA1-mutation carriers. Breast cancer linkage consortium. Am J Hum Genet 1995;56: 265–71.

82. Collaborative Group on Hormonal Factors in Breast Cancer. Familial breast cancer: collaborative reanalysis of individual data from 52 epidemiological studies including 58,209 women with breast cancer and 101,986 women without the disease. Lancet 2001;358:1389–99.
83. Petrucelli N, Daly MB, Culver JOB, et al. BRCA1 and BRCA2 hereditary breast/ovarian cancer. Gene reviews. Available at: http://www.genetests.org/querydz=brcal. Accessed January 5, 2010.
84. Amir E, Evans DG, Shenton A, et al. Evaluation of breast cancer risk assessment packages in the family history evaluation and screening programme. J Med Genet 2003;40:807–14.
85. Fisher B, Anderson S, Redmond CK, et al. Reanalysis and results after 12 years of follow-up in a randomized clinical trial comparing total mastectomy with lumpectomy with or without irradiation in the treatment of breast cancer. N Engl J Med 1995;333:1456–61.
86. Fisher B, Anderson S, Bryant J, et al. Twenty-year follow-up of a randomized trial comparing total mastectomy, lumpectomy, and lumpectomy plus irradiation for the treatment of invasive breast cancer. N Engl J Med 2002;347:1233–41.
87. Easton DF. Familial risks of breast cancer. Breast Cancer Res 2002;4:179–81.
88. Frykberg ER. Lobular carcinoma in situ of the breast. Breast J 1999;5:296–303.
89. Dupont WD, Parl FF, Hartmann WH, et al. Breast cancer risk associated with proliferative breast disease and atypical hyperplasia. Cancer 1993;71:1258–65.
90. Page DL, Schuyler PA, Dupont WD, et al. Atypical lobular hyperplasia as a unilateral predictor of breast cancer risk: a retrospective cohort study. Lancet 2003; 361:125–9.
91. Boyd NE, Guo H, Martin LJ, et al. Mammographic density and the risk and detection of breast cancer. N Engl J Med 2007;356:227–36.
92. Berg WA. Tailored supplementary screening for breast cancer: what now and what next? AJR Am J Roentgenol 2009;192:390–9.
93. Hendrick RE. Breast MRI: fundamental and technical aspects. New York: Springer Verlag; 2008.
94. La Trenta LR, Menell JH, Morris EA, et al. Breast lesions detected with MR imaging: utility and histopathologic importance of identification with US. Radiology 2003;227:856–61.
95. Feig SA, Shaber GS, Patchefsky A, et al. Analysis of clinically and mammographically occult breast tumors. AJR Am J Roentgenol 1977;128:403–8.
96. Kerlikowske K, Grady D, Barclay J, et al. Effect of age, breast density, and family history on the sensitivity of first screening mammography. JAMA 1996; 276:33–8.
97. Rosenberg RD, Hunt WC, Williamson MR, et al. Effects of age, breast density, ethnicity, and estrogen replacement therapy on screening mammographic sensitivity and cancer stage at diagnosis: review of 183, 134 screening mammograms in Albuquerque, New Mexico. Radiology 1998;209:511–8.
98. van Gils CH, Otten JD, Verbeeck AL, et al. Effect of mammographic breast density on breast cancer screening performance: a study in Nijmegen, the Netherlands. J Epidemiol Community Health 1998;52:267–71.
99. Mandelson MT, Oestreicher N, Porter PL, et al. Breast density as a predictor of mammographic detection: comparison of interval and screen-detected cancers. J Natl Cancer Inst 2000;92:1081–7.
100. Ma I, Fischell C, Wright B, et al. Case control study of factors associated with failure to detect breast cancer by mammography. J Natl Cancer Inst 2000;92: 1081–7.

101. Jackson VP, Hendrick RE, Feig SA, et al. Imaging the radiographically dense breast. Radiology 1993;188:297–301.
102. Stomper PC, D'Souza DJ, DiNitto PA, et al. Analysis of parenchymal density on mammograms of 1353 women 25–79 years old. AJR Am J Roentgenol 1996; 167:1261–5.
103. Gordon PB, Goldenberg SL. Malignant breast masses detected only by ultrasound: a retrospective review. Cancer 1995;76:626–30.
104. Kolb TM, Lichy J, Newhouse JH. Occult cancer in women with dense breast: detection with screening US-diagnostic yield and tumor characteristics. Radiology 1998;207:191–9.
105. Buchberger W, DeKoekkoek-Doll P, Springer P, et al. Incidental findings on sonography of the breast clinical significance and diagnostic workup. AJR Am J Roentgenol 1999;173:921–7.
106. Buchberger W, Niehoff A, Orbist A, et al. Clinically and mammographically occult breast lesions; detection and classification with high-resolution sonography. Semin Ultrasound CT MR 2000;21:325–36.
107. Kaplan SS. Clinical utility of bilateral whole-breast US in the evaluation of women with dense breast tissue. Radiology 2001;221:641–9.
108. Kolb TM, Lichy J, Newhouse JH. Comparison of the performance of screening mammography physical examination, and breast US and evaluation of factors that influence them: an analysis of 27,825 patient evaluation. Radiology 2002; 225:165–75.
109. Leconte I, Feger C, Galant C, et al. Mammography and subsequent whole-breast sonography of nonpalpable breast cancers: the importance of radiologic breast density. AJR Am J Roentgenol 2003;180:1675–9.
110. Crystal P, Strano S, Shcharynski S, et al. Using sonography to screen women with mammographically dense breasts. AJR Am J Roentgenol 2003;181: 177–82.
111. Feig SA. Current status of screening US. Breast imaging: RSNA categorical course in diagnostic radiology. Oak Brook (IL): Radiological Society of North America Inc; 2005. p. 143–54.
112. Bassett LW, Hendrick RE, Bassford TL, et al. Clinical practice guideline number 13: quality determinants of mammography. AHCPR Publication 95-0632. Rockville (MD): US Department of Health and Human Services, Agency for Health Care Policy and Research, Public Health Service; 1994. p. 83.
113. Feig SA. Auditing and benchmarks in screening and diagnostic mammography. Radiol Clin North Am 2007;45:791–800.
114. Berg WA, Blume JD, Cormack JB, et al. Combined screening with ultrasound and mammography versus mammography alone in women at elevated risk of breast cancer. JAMA 2008;299(18):2151–63.
115. Corsetti V, Houssami N, Ferrari A, et al. Breast screening with ultrasound in women with mammography-negative dense breasts: evidence on incremental cancer detection and false positives, and associated cost. Eur J Cancer 2008;44:539–44.
116. Enzmann DR, Anglada PM, Haviley C, et al. Providing professional mammography services: financial analysis. Radiology 2001;219:467–73.
117. Chou YH, Tiu C-M, Chen J, et al. Automated full-field breast ultrasonography: the past and the present. J Med Ultrasound 2007;15(1):31–44.
118. Kelly KM, Dean J, Comulada WS, et al. Breast cancer detection using automated whole breast ultrasound and mammography in radiographically dense breasts. Eur Radiol 2010;20:734–42.

Index

Note: Page numbers of article titles are in **boldface** type.

Obstet Gynecol Clin N Am 38 (2011) 197–204
doi:10.1016/S0889-8545(11)00010-6
0889-8545/11/$ – see front matter © 2011 Elsevier Inc. All rights reserved.

obgyn.theclinics.com

Moving?

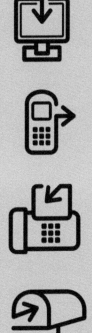

Printed and bound by CPI Group (UK) Ltd, Croydon, CR0 4YY

03/10/2024

01040457-0019

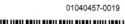